HANDS HEAL:
DOCUMENTATION FOR MASSAGE THERAPY

A guide to SOAP charting

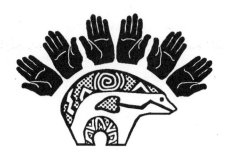

by Diana L. Thompson, L.M.P.

HANDS HEAL: DOCUMENTATION FOR MASSAGE THERAPY
A Guide to SOAP Charting

by Diana L. Thompson, L.M.P.

Edited by Phoenix

Graphic Design by Jackie A. Phillips

Cover art by Debra Bacianga

First Printing July 1993
Printed in the United States of America
Copyright © 1993 by Diana L. Thompson
Published by Diana L. Thompson, Seattle, Washington

ISBN 0-9638347-0-3

For information write:
Diana L. Thompson, L.M.P.
Healing Arts Studio
916 N.E. 64th
Seattle, Washington 98115

PRINTED ON
RECYCLED PAPER

Table of Contents

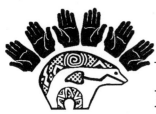

Introduction

HOW I CAME TO WRITE THIS BOOK

My personal experience of SOAP charting began in 1986 when I was performing massage therapy out of the chiropractic offices of Dr. Lisanne Yuricich and Dr. Manda Rae Davis in Seattle. I had been licensed to do massage since January 1984, but had been primarily treating sports injuries. Then, in 1985, I was involved in a motor vehicle accident and experienced the value of massage treatment for the resulting injuries. Upon my recovery, I began treating acute traumatic injuries on a full-time basis.

I learned quickly that insurance companies required chart notes to substantiate claims. Attorney Richard Adler taught me the basic legal requirements of such documentation, and recommended that I use SOAP charting. His workshops and my access to chiropractors' charts on our mutual clients comprised my only initial resources for learning the technique.

In 1987 I opened and practiced at Lakeside Massage, an injury clinic which quickly grew to support a staff of fifteen massage therapists. Drawing on our collective experiences, I developed a system of SOAP charting specific to the massage treatment of injuries.

Later in 1987 I began teaching this charting system to massage therapists in local workshops on insurance billings and practice management for personal injury cases. Soon after, I began lecturing on the subject at American Massage Therapy Association (AMTA) conventions in Oregon and Washington, and at Northwest Massage Practitioners Association (NWMPA) professional series. By 1990 I was teaching SOAP charting at several massage schools in western Washington.

I saw the need to develop a more general SOAP format for massage therapists when I began teaching full-time at the Seattle Massage School. I realized that charting had a broader application than documentation for insurance companies, that it is a valuable tool for all types and applications of massage therapy. So, with the assistance of the clinical team and hundreds of students, and with the permission of the board of Seattle Massage School, I have developed the system you will find in this book: *Hands Heal—Documentation for Massage Therapy.*

ACKNOWLEDGE-MENTS

To Annie Thoe, the energetic creative genius behind every SOAP chart revision, I owe my deepest gratitude.

I sincerely thank the hundreds of massage students who were forced to be flexible, adapting to a "new and improved" revision of charting quarter after quarter. Without your feedback this book would not have been possible.

Without Lisanne Yuricich and Richard Adler I would still be attending the school of hard knocks. Thank you for your kind and gentle teachings.

Kerry Ann Plunkett, Dawn Schmidt and everyone at Seattle Massage School provided me the freedom to grow. Thank you for your trust.

Phoenix and Debra Bacianga turned my ideas into art. Thank you for your hard work and creative spirit.

Thank you Jackie for your support, encouragement and inspiration. You have this amazing ability to breathe life into letters on a page, and into me. You are a brilliant designer. I love you.

To all of you who have contributed to this process, THANK YOU!! Barb Frye, Clint Chandler, Adam Bailey, Sarah Contreras, Susan Cowley-Head, Dee Spath, my many illustrious T.A.'s, Manda Rae Davis, my former staff at Lakeside, Barb Collins of Spectrum Massage School, Brian Utting's School of Massage, all of my students, my clients, my teachers, Sage Reed, Kerric and Matthew, Sheila and Bill W., my spiritual support from my mother and grandparents, the inner strength of Bear spirit and the guiding light of Moon spirit.

Thank you to all participants in hands-on healing. I wish you health and prosperity.

DEDICATION

In memory of Kirshe, Nikki and Ivar–the animals spirits who have blessed my earthly existence.

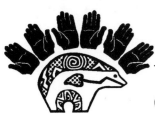

Chapter 1: *What Is SOAP Charting?*

SOAP—Subjective Objective Assessment Plan—charting is a popular format for documenting treatment sessions in the health care field, routinely used by chiropractors, physical therapists, doctors, and nurses. The purpose of a SOAP chart is to document the client's history and current complaints, the practitioner's findings and treatment, changes resulting from treatment, and guidelines for the client and for future treatments. An increasing number of massage curriculums across the country are including SOAP charting as the standard format for documenting massage sessions. Any massage style or technique can be documented thoroughly and easily due to the flexibility and simple structure of the SOAP format.

In brief, a chart is composed of:

> SUBJECTIVE information—what the client tells you about health history and current symptoms;

> OBJECTIVE information—your observations and the results of the tests you perform;

> ASSESSMENT—changes in the client's condition as a result of treatment; and

> PLAN—suggested future treatment.

WHO BENEFITS FROM THIS INFORMATION?

The Licensed Massage Practitioner (LMP), the primary caregiver, and the client all benefit from this information.

The LMP must be aware of client history and progress in order to make appropriate treatment decisions.

The primary caregiver must be informed of the LMP's soft tissue findings, treatment modalities, and client progress in order to make educated decisions regarding continuing massage care.

Clients can be regularly informed of progress through SOAP charting and can become more active participants in their own healing process.

The charting process builds a bridge between your client, yourself and other health care providers.

In addition, documentation through SOAP charting protects all those involved from legal problems. In many states, licensed health care providers are legally required to document treatments both for health maintenance and for injuries. And in the event of personal injury insurance litigation, documentation is always required. The client's records may be subpoenaed as evidence of significant injury and as proof of reasonable and necessary care for your financial reimbursement. If your records are good, you can avoid going to court to defend them.

SOAP charting is being widely adopted by massage professionals for several reasons:

1. Other health care professionals find the format and language familiar, providing an essential communication tool.

2. Use of a professional reporting system enhances the image of massage as a valuable therapy.

3. Charting validates massage as curative adjunctive treatment by proving client progress.

4. It is accepted by insurance companies as proof of reasonable and necessary care.

5. It provides evidence for attorneys as proof of significant injury.

6. It suggests a structure for potential research using case studies.

SOAP charting is an efficient, effective way to document all types of health care treatment. Writing SOAP charts is good business and good for business.

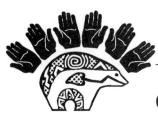

Chapter 2: *Subjective Information*

WHAT IS SUBJECTIVE INFORMATION?

All the things a client **tells** you come under the heading of subjective information. This includes the client's previous history, present symptoms, any aggravating circumstances or changes in activity due to the existing symptoms, anything the client has found that relieves the symptoms, and a description of the onset or initial cause of the symptoms. Much of the information may be obtained through Medical History or Intake Forms and Pain Questionnaires. The rest will be obtained by interview, and recorded on the SOAP chart.

WHY ARE WE INTERESTED IN SUBJECTIVE INFORMATION?

We gather subjective information for three reasons. The first is that through exploring their physical sensations, clients learn to listen to their bodies' needs and signals. By describing their physical sensations and their feelings about them, they establish or strengthen a mind/body connection. This connection is often weak and may even seem at times nonexistent, particularly in people living with chronic pain. Clients' symptoms may be so uncomfortable that they disassociate from their bodies. They become unable to hear their bodies' warning signals. Encouraging this mind/body connection through questioning and consulting clients about their physical and emotional concerns and goals gives them an opportunity to identify their bodies' needs, to chose how and when those needs may be met, and to participate actively in their healing process. Assist a person to establish a relationship with her body and you give her back the power to take care of herself.

Secondly, the more physical or emotional data we can identify by documenting symptoms, the more we can justify treating the body as a whole. More often than not, the initial imbalance becomes a syndrome, a complication of multiple dysfunctions, and involves the entire body. The initial trauma can lead to complicating compensational holding patterns that often become a larger problem than the original injury. Through the discovery of the connecting symptoms we can document the interrelatedness of the body and address the whole person, rather than concentrating on treating the initial problem. Too often insurance companies insist that only the injured site receive treatment. If properly documented, treatment to the associated structures is reimbursable.

Proving progress

Thirdly, the more specific the information documented, the greater the possibility of noting change as a result of the massage treatment. Comparing the differences in symptoms before and after the massage demonstrates the effectiveness of the treatment. This validates massage as a viable treatment modality and encourages clients to chose massage for their adjunctive health care. Many massage modalities are easy to incorporate into daily living. When shown how effective it can be, many clients will incorporate self-care, like hydrotherapy, stretching, and self-massage, into their personal care routines. Educating people in self-care is a responsibility of all health care providers.

In addition, thorough documentation of subjective information contributes to substantiating significant injury. In insurance disputes, your care must be proven "reasonable and necessary" to insure payment to you, or reimbursement to the client. Many insurance companies will not pay for maintenance health care. "Reasonable and necessary" is the term used to validate a treatment modality. If reasonable cause (proof of significant injury) and success of treatment (a decrease in symptoms) can be substantiated, the care is considered curative not palliative.-*just comforting*

MEDICAL HISTORY/ INTAKE FORMS

Intake forms gather specific data regarding the client's past. They contain a series of standard health questions about circulatory problems, respiratory problems, diseases, infections, medications, surgeries, accidents and activity levels. A medical history will help establish if there are indications and contraindications for massage treatment. Discuss any contraindications with your client and determine if a doctor's permission is necessary for treatment, or if certain areas or treatment techniques should be avoided. Knowledge of these pre-existing conditions is also important in determining pre-injury status and liability in insurance cases. Intake forms may also provide information regarding clients' familiarity with massage, their likes and dislikes regarding treatment styles and their comfort levels for touch.

The intake forms consist of the following:

1. PERSONAL HEALTH INFORMATION, which includes:
    - Personal data
    - Massage history and treatment information
    - Health history
    - Disclaimer with client signature
    Note: This form is updated annually.

2. PERSONAL STATUS FORM, which includes:
    - Figures on which client draws symptoms
    - A key defining the symbols the client uses in drawing symptoms
    Note: This form is updated with each status report.

3. INJURY INFORMATION INTAKE, which includes:
    - Description of onset
    - Symptoms:
        -current
        -immediate post-injury
        -all other symptoms prior to date of initial treatment
    - Necessary physical activities
    - Aggravating activities of daily living
    - Adjunctive therapies

- Insurance and attorney information
- Billing information

Note: This form is completed only once, for the initial visit.

4. OSWESTRY / VERNON/MIOR PAIN QUESTIONNAIRE, which includes:
   - Rating activities of daily living affected by back pain
   - Rating activities of daily living affected by neck pain

Note: This form can be updated weekly, or just at status report sessions.

You may choose to save time by sending out your intake forms in the mail prior to the first session. People often breeze through the forms in the office because they are eager to get on with the session. When given their own time to really think about the questions, to look things up if necessary, or to ask family members for help in reconstructing events, their information tends to be more complete. Occasionally people do forget to bring the forms to the initial visit, but the majority remember and make it worth the trouble of doing the advance mailing.

Before you begin the first massage session, go over the intake forms with your client. It gives you a starting point for your subjective information gathering and helps you qualify current symptoms and patient complaints. Detailed information also enables you to do a thorough objective search involving viewing, palpating and testing the appropriate areas, which will result in streamlined, efficient treatment. This will produce the best results and will help in designing future treatment plans.

PAIN QUESTIONNAIRES

Pain questionnaires are effective ways to document how symptoms are affecting activities of daily living. Insurance companies have begun to rely on them to determine when clients may return to work, and to establish compensation for their injuries. Increasingly, these companies recognize that a return to full-time work does not mean that the client is completely recovered, so they consider other factors as well, such as ability to resume pre-injury household tasks, child care, hobbies, and personal activities. There are several forms available for this purpose, but the Oswestry / Vernon/Mior pain questionnaire is the most detailed I have found to date. These forms may be completed weekly or be reserved for status report sessions.

INTERVIEWING SKILLS

Interviewing is an information-gathering process. Your client possesses all the information you need; you must simply learn to ask the correct questions and listen carefully to the replies. The clearer the questions, the more specific the answers. Elicit the most detailed picture possible, both to document dysfunction and, ultimately, to show progress or change due to treatment.

Remember too that sometimes the process of asking questions and gathering subjective information itself can be far more important than identifying a cause or pinpointing a dysfunction, since it can lead a client to a better understanding of the interrelation of body systems and of the mind-body connection.

The primary skill in interviewing is **listening**. Careful listening will not only yield information, but will indicate directions for further questions. Attentive, respectful listening and follow-up questions will help build a relationship of trust and cooperation that will insure obtaining the most complete picture.

LISTENING SKILLS

An examiner for a doctoral program in neurology explains that over half their candidates fail the oral exams, largely, he thinks, because they don't listen to everything the patient is saying and therefore don't obtain adequate information. They are too apt to focus on listening for a key phrase or word that points to a familiar dysfunction. Instead, he says, they should pursue lines of questioning suggested by the client's comments and gather more information on which to base their conclusions.

Massage practitioners also must avoid the temptation to jump too quickly to conclusions about the cause of a client's symptoms. Don't overlook important compensational or secondary symptoms. Remember that hypomobility in one joint leads to hypermobility of another, that a postural adaptation to pain leads to a compensational postural adaptation someplace else. Being thorough in your investigation will lead to a more thorough treatment. It may also keep you from diagnosis, which is outside the scope of practice of massage.

LEADING QUESTIONS

The second component of good interviewing skills is the ability to ask leading questions. A good interviewer learns to pick the significant details out of a client's story and to listen for clues which provide a direction for further questions. You must learn to stay on track and not be distracted by irrelevant detail or by personal information.

Leading questions direct the client to give the specific types of information desired, and spur the memory to uncover more data. This may involve inquiring about repetitive actions in the client's work, home and play activities to explain a possible gradual onset repetitive movement injury. Often clients only look for an obvious cause, for something they did differently that resulted in injury. But gradual onset injuries involve things they did in the same way, day after day. Try questions like:

"Do you sit, stand, or lift a lot at work?"
"Do you often carry your portfolio/purse/backpack on the same shoulder?"
"Do you usually cross the same leg?"
"Do you talk on the phone a lot?"

Learn to follow a line of thought. If a client reports low back pain, you might ask how her knees have been lately, or if he has occasional numbness and tingling down his leg. Symptoms are generally related to other symptoms; one leads to another. Rarely is a symptom an isolated phenomenon, especially in a chronic situation. The body compensates in so many ways to attempt to maintain a balance that it is essential to explore all possibilities.

Familiarity with common soft tissue dysfunctions and with the relationship of body and movement will suggest productive lines of inquiry.

Leading questions also impose consistency on descriptions of symptoms. Prompt the client with adjectives like *mild*, *moderate*, or *severe* when you ask them to describe their pain. Using consistent terminology to describe a symptom will show progress or change more clearly. It is easier to compare the progress from "moderate pain" to "mild pain" than trying to distinguish between "hurts pretty bad" to "kinda sore". The ability to prove progress is an important component of documenting information.

Acquiring information from your client is an art. You will need to cultivate a flexible style to accommodate your clients' differences in background and in knowledge about massage therapy and other health matters. It is important to use language that your client understands, yet still use consistent terminology. As you ask your questions, simply define any specialized terms that you use as a matter of course. Avoid both speaking down to clients and speaking over their heads.

COMMON PROBLEMS

Of course, it will not always be easy to elicit the information you need.

Some clients will initially report no pain, no symptoms. Many chronic pain sufferers, for example, have developed very high pain tolerances. Other clients may have become desensitized to their bodies, but during the massage will discover sore or tight spots and will begin to remember all the accidents and injuries they had previously forgotten. Symptoms from those old injuries may recur periodically, perhaps in times of stress or after unusually strenuous activities.

You will also find clients who seem to have difficulty talking about their pain or their bodily functions. Looking at their drawings on the intake forms, their medical histories, and their stated goals may suggest questions to ask. Sometimes they find discussing their problems uncomfortable, but have no trouble putting the information on a drawing. The difficulty may lie in your choice of language. Try substituting other words in your questions—ask about "tension" or "tightness" rather than "pain" or "dysfunction", for example. Be flexible in your approach and vocabulary; do not expect the client to make the adjustment.

Other clients may be too verbose, and will offer more detail than you need. Often they will give their information in a disjointed fashion, with discussion of one symptom leading to recollection of another injury, which reminds them of more details about a previously discussed symptom. Fortunately, when you record this on a structured chart you can skip around, yet still be sure your information is complete.

Another common problem is that people often mention only the pain that is prominent at a given moment. When they report pain the next week in a totally different location, it is generally treated as a new symptom. It is likely, however, that it was present but less prominent all along.

Here are some suggestions for difficult situations:

Steer clients away from giving too much personal information during questioning. It's important to know about events and situations that affect your clients' health, but not necessary or appropriate to know all the details. You would want to know, for example, that your client was feeling stressed by financial pressures; you don't need to hear about her second mortgage, her children's college bills, or her VISA balance.

Help your clients describe their symptoms by prompting them with certain consistent adjectives. Qualify the information using descriptive adjectives in order to note progress accurately in the future. It is important to feed your client descriptive words to maintain consistency. For example, ask:
"Is your arm pain *mild, moderate* or *severe*?"
"Does your head ache *constantly, intermittently* or *seldom*?"

Ask about symptoms that aren't prominent at the moment. Find out, for example, what symptoms the client has experienced off and on since a car accident. If the client reports elbow pain, ask if he also has numbness and tingling in the hand, or neck pain or stiffness. If the client isn't experiencing pain at that time, ask when and where she commonly does feel it. Where does he usually hold his stress? How long was she in a cast? Did he walk with crutches for a long time?

Stick to three primary symptoms each session. Only at status report sessions do you have time to cover all the symptoms.

Three symptoms may be difficult for some people to come up with. Check their intake forms for previous injuries that may present themselves on occasion. People often report that they are only receiving massage to relax. Explore their tension-holding patterns to uncover possible symptoms. They may not be experiencing any symptoms today, so inquire about where they do hold tension when they are experiencing stress and physical discomfort. If they seem eager to get on with the massage, gently question them as you discover hypertonicities, trigger points, or adhesions in their body during the massage.

Remember, though, that "three symptoms per session" is just a guideline, a maximum number to treat. We do not want to create symptoms when there are none; we just want to be thorough.

Information gathering does not end once they get on the table. With care, you can continue throughout the massage and still fulfill the client's request for relaxation. Additional information will always trickle in. As it does, add it to your intake form, initial it and date it.

DOCUMENTING INFORMATION

Subjective information may be documented by using the client's own words in quotes, or by paraphrasing. A mix of both is most effective. Clients often say powerful things regarding their feelings that should be preserved in quotes. However, for the sake of consistency, speed and efficiency, most information should be paraphrased, using consistent descriptive terms. You will find examples of these terms throughout the following text.

In addition, medical abbreviations are a useful shorthand. You will find a list of common medical abbreviations that relate to the practice of massage in the Appendix. Become familiar with these, and add any others that you find useful. Use them consistently, and be sure to include a copy with your SOAP charts whenever your charts are requested.

TIMING

Your goal in the interview is to gather a general medical history and a complete picture of the client's current symptoms and physical complaints. Plenty of time should be allotted for this process. Explain this in advance to your clients so that they know exactly what to expect. You may need an additional half hour for the initial interview as well as the hour of treatment time.

The initial interview process can be time-consuming. To speed up the charting, use abbreviations as often as possible.

Use this interview time to get an idea of your clients' relationship with their bodies. Familiarize yourself with their level of body awareness, their expectations, and set short and long term goals with them regarding the massage sessions, their progress and their activities of daily living. Discuss their commitment to participate in their health care and educate them about massage techniques and treatment choices.

Try to do a complete interview during the first session or two rather than having information trickling in over the course of treatment. You will save time; you may save much more than time. Consider the poor student whose client told her at the **end** of a massage session that she had a blood clot in her neck. She'd forgotten to mention it on her intake form. A thorough interview might have jogged her memory and removed the possibility of a life-endangering incident.

Communication is what interviewing is about. Listen to your clients' needs and respond to them, document them and their response. Your massage relationship is based on open, honest, constant communication. The effectiveness of your massages will improve as a result of improving your communication skills and interviewing skills.

WHAT GOES ON THE CHART

With just a client's intake forms, one could go on to establish the client's goals for the immediate session, determine any contraindications to massage, and devise a plan or approach for a safe massage session.

Much more subjective information is required in a superior SOAP chart, however. You will also need to elicit more detailed information about their physical symptoms and the emotional complications resulting from the symptoms, about how these symptoms are affecting their ability to function in life, and about activities of daily living that may aggravate or relieve the symptoms. These are all subjective data.

Subjective information also includes anything else clients tell you. Responses to the last session may be included, as may reported information from primary caregivers regarding diagnosis of previous or current conditions, past or present treatment modalities for those conditions, or anything else that clients know to be true regarding their well-being.

CLIENT GOALS

The primary concern of every massage practitioner is to hear the current needs of the client and to design each session to meet those needs. Often we have agendas based on what we think is best for our clients. We may see things that need "fixing" and be eager to impress our clients with our ability to treat their conditions. People's bodies seem to be capable of preventing change when change is unwanted or unprepared for. Therefore the session should begin by identifying the **clients'** needs and goals.

Common responses from clients regarding their goals include:
"I just want to relax."
"Can you get rid of this pain?"
"I only want my back rubbed."
"I want to go back to running again—fix my knee, please."

You will also frequently hear statements like:
"I don't know how to relax."
"Watch out—my feet are ticklish."

All of these statements contain messages that need to be addressed. It is important to communicate further with the client to discover more information.

"I just want to relax" usually indicates tension or muscle-guarding in one or more areas. Ask the client for more specifics. For example, does he experience tension in any particular part of his body? Would she like to decrease tightness in any specific muscles or increase movement in any particular joint? These questions encourage clients to scan their bodies and listen to any signals regarding physical discomfort. This is a great way to bring possible problem areas into awareness and to connect the mind-body communication system. This awareness also provides an opportunity to demonstrate the effectiveness of the session when re-evaluating posture and movement.

"I don't know how to relax" opens an avenue for the practitioner to increase the client's awareness of his body and relationship to his environment. Here it is important not to tell clients to "relax" during a massage, or to scold them for not letting go. Use gentle cues like "let your arm feel heavy" instead of a command like "relax your arm". Create a context for the body to remember what it feels like to be relaxed, using verbal instructions like "this is what it feels like to be relaxed. You can return to this state at any time simply by recalling this feeling". It is easier for the body to deal with stress when it is aware of when it is stressed and what that feels like. Use these opportunities to educate clients and increase their awareness whenever possible.

Help your client to create attainable goals. Suggest that "decreasing the pain" or "increasing the function" are more realistic goals than "stop the pain" or "fix the knee". Don't foster the expectation that you can perform swift or complete cures. Instead, try to encourage an atmosphere of teamwork and client participation.

When clients mention that they are ticklish or say that they just want their back rubbed, it may indicate an uneasiness about being touched. It is important here to be sensitive to touch issues and practice a "safe touch protocol". (You might want to read Clyde Ford's *Where Healing Waters Meet* to learn more about "safe touch".) Respect their wishes and ask if there are certain body parts that they do not want massaged; let them know this is a common and acceptable request. Indicate that the client has a right at all times to stop treatment on any particular part of their body, and encourage them to express any needs in order to feel comfortable and safe. Complete information on your draping procedure and a play-by-play preview of the treatment plan for the day may be helpful in easing any nervous tension and avoiding unmet expectations.

Under client goals you might also include types of massage that clients liked or disliked and want included or excluded from their massage session. Ask if there are particular parts of the body that they want you to concentrate on. Ask if they would prefer lotion or oil. Before the massage begins, encourage clients to feel free to ask for more or less of anything—depth of pressure, a particular technique, or information about what you are doing, at any time during the massage. Remind them that this is their massage and it is your intention to meet their needs and goals whenever possible. Put them at ease as much as possible before they even get on the table. Chart what works.

UPDATE

Update symptoms by noting the clients' response to the last session. This demonstrates the effect the treatment had on the client and may contribute to client and treatment goals. For example, head ache decreased in severity for three days post treatment. (Abbreviation: HA ↓ 3 dys post tx)

SYMPTOMS

As massage therapists we cannot diagnose physical conditions or the emotional well-being of a client. It is to our advantage therefore to elicit as much information as possible from the client to document dysfunction, rather than relying solely on the information we can uncover through visual and palpable observations.

Physical symptoms may include pain or discomfort, tightness or stiffness, loss of function or mobility, fatigue or irregular sleep patterns, poor posture, numbness and tingling, cramping or muscle spasms, to name a few.

Emotional complications often include depression, anxiety and stress. When dealing with insurance cases, it is crucial to relate the emotional symptoms to the physical symptoms. For example, a client might complain of depression because her back pain prevents her from picking up her infant as often as they both would like. If you fail to make this cause-effect relationship clear, the insurance company may red flag the case and attempt to cut off care due to unstable character, or potential for malingering.

Emotional components can only be documented as subjective symptoms, not as objective findings, within the scope of practice of massage practitioners. Emotional symptoms are valid, however, and should be included. New research is finding that the function of the immune system is heavily influenced by our emotional states. In many cases we don't know which came first, the emotional or the physical imbalance. In either case, massage can improve and support the healing process.

It's important to gather symptoms even in the absence of personal injury or specific trauma. Those clients who present themselves for a massage reporting that they are fine and simply in need of a relaxing massage often have unconscious body imbalances. Most people in need of relaxation suffer from stresses of daily living. Because of the body's ability to manifest emotions physically, the body exhibits signs of stress in the form of tight muscles, postural adaptations, depressed immune systems and visceral dysfunctions. Poor posture, fatigue, indigestion, constipation and headaches are common results of stress. When these go untreated, physical injuries occur on subtle levels. These may advance into repetitive movement injuries like carpal tunnel or thoracic outlet syndrome, or into serious health problems like high blood pressure or cancer.

Subjective data obtained for relaxation massage can document simple stress warning signs like tight muscles, fatigue and poor posture. This may increase the client's awareness of these symptoms. Receiving relaxation massage can assist people in learning to deal with stress and take better care of themselves. Providing education on self-care can help people help themselves. Simple life changes, such as one-sided movements being shared and evened out, or repetitive movements being interrupted by breaks and stretching, can end a vicious cycle. We can assist people by strengthening that mind-body connection and by treating the whole person. Preventive health care is the cheapest form of health care. SOAP charting is an easy, effective way to bring awareness to imbalances in the body that may develop into serious health problems.

SYMPTOM LOCATION, INTENSITY, DURATION, FREQUENCY, and ONSET

Once you've obtained a symptom, it must be qualified. *Location, intensity, duration* and *frequency* provide sufficient information for noting progress. Without qualification, it would be difficult to differentiate the client's status from session to session.

Consider the following example:

A client presents herself complaining of a headache. She receives a massage, feels better—no more headache—and goes her merry way. Same client is back in a week complaining of a headache. She receives a massage, feels better—no more headache—and goes her merry way. This happens for four weeks without change. The massage practitioner feels inadequate and begins waiting tables with his extra time instead of marketing.

An improved scenario:

A client presents herself complaining of a headache. The massage practitioner questions the client further and discovers that the headache is behind both eyes, is moderately painful and has been constant for three weeks. The client receives a massage, feels better —no more headache—and goes her merry way. Same client is back in week complaining of a headache. The practitioner questions her further and discovers that the headache pain is behind both eyes, is moderate in pain but better than last week, has occurred daily for the past week, lasting about 3-4 hours each time. She receives a massage, feels better—no more headache—and goes her merry way. The next visit her symptoms include mild headache pain behind the left eye, occurring bi-weekly, lasting for 3-4 hours. The next week her symptoms include mild headache pain behind her left eye, occurring twice that week, with a duration of 2 hours. The next week her symptoms include mild headache pain behind the left eye, and this is her first headache all week and began when she got stuck in traffic on her way to her massage appointment.

The massage practitioner runs out to medical clinics in the area to market for headache patients, flaunting the SOAP charts proving progress, with the client's name carefully whited out for confidentiality.

LOCATION

The exact location of a symptom can aid in clear documentation and efficient treatment of the symptom. Janet Travell states in her book *Myofascial Pain and Dysfunction* that the specific location of headache pain can identify the muscle in need of trigger point therapy. If, for example, the headache is located in the forehead over the left eye, the trigger point can most likely be found in the left sternocleidomastoid. If someone is complaining of low back pain it is helpful to know if that area denotes the thoraco-lumbar junction, the lumbo-sacral junction or the sacro-iliac junction. Identifying the specific location of the symptom clearly documents the dysfunction and allows for fast, efficient and effective treatment.

Clarity in location provides clearer opportunities to demonstrate the relationship between the initial dysfunction and compensatory adaptations. It is important to remember to treat the whole person and not to focus narrowly on the initial injury or symptom.

INTENSITY

The intensity of a symptom can be qualified on a simple three point scale using *mild* or *light*, *moderate* and *severe* as the descriptive terms. This is less complicated than a scale of one to ten, which is subject to variable interpretations. It can easily be transformed into a nine point scale by simply adding a plus or a minus to each when slight changes are important to note. These may be abbreviated with L, M, S or L-, L, L+, M-, M, M+, S-, S, S+. Be conservative regarding your use of severe; save it for your worst case scenarios.

DURATION

Duration denotes how long the symptom lasts when it occurs. This may be described using seconds, minutes, hours, days, weeks, months, or years. These are easily abbreviated by dropping the vowels or shortening the words. (Sec., min., hrs., dys., wks., mths., yrs.)

FREQUENCY

Frequency describes how often the symptom occurs. Standard adjectives to describe how often include *seldom, intermittent, frequent,* and *constant.* Abbreviations for these are seld., inter., freq., and cons. Or you might use more specific descriptions, like twice a week, three times a day, hourly, monthly, etc. Abbreviations might include 2x/wk, 3x/dy, hrly, mthly.

DESCRIPTION OF ONSET

Description of onset documents the biomechanics of the body positions and movements involved in the injury as well as external conditions affecting the injury. Describing the biomechanics of a lift-and-twist injury, for example, requires identifying the side of the body moving the weight, and the direction the body was turning in order to accurately determine which muscles are being over-stretched and which muscles are over-contracting. In the case of a fall, it is important to note what body parts contacted what type of surface and in what order. This information helps determine appropriate treatment and streamlines the sessions to meet each individual's needs.

Also included in onset is the length of time this symptom has been occurring. For example, perhaps the client suffered from a motor vehicle accident on April 15, 1992. Both the date and the cause of the onset are important.

In the case of a repetitive movement injury, the onset would need to include the action that was being repeated over and over and to describe any other important data. For example:

> Hammers repeatedly at shoulder height with right hand, 15 pound hammer, 8 hours/day, 5 days/week, 5 years at job, carrying nail pouch on left hip.

The date of the onset may be difficult to determine in this scenario. Find out from the client the approximate year the symptoms began. Determine a month if possible, or a time of year. "Summer of 42", or "December 83" is more informative than "for years".

In the case of a traumatic whiplash injury, the description of onset would include many external factors as well, including the size of the vehicles, the weather conditions, the speed and direction of impact, the use of seat belts, the position of the headrests, and whether the vehicle was at rest or in motion. The physical mechanisms involved include the position of the head at the time of impact, whether hyperflexion or hyperextension was the initial action, if rotation was involved. (For more details, see *Medical-Legal Aspects of Soft Tissue Injury*, by Richard Adler, or *Whiplash Injuries–The Cervical Acceleration/Deceleration Syndrom*, by Forman and Croft)

It is not uncommon to have an insurance company challenge the necessity of treatment. Often Labor and Industries only permits treatment on the injury itself. Having a clear understanding of the mechanisms of the injury will help justify treating a broader area. For example, with a lift-and-twist injury the diagnosis may be a low back sprain/strain. Treatment to the neck and shoulders may seem luxurious and unnecessary to an insurance adjuster unless you can clearly explain the biomechanical linkages and compensating symptoms involved.

The initial status report or intake form should document the specific details of the onset. A brief account of the information can be included on the daily SOAP charts as a reminder.

AGGRAVATING AND RELIEVING CIRCUMSTANCES

In documenting significant injury and in noting progress it's important to record the circumstances encountered in the course of daily living that seem to aggravate or relieve symptoms. This gives both practitioner and client a frame of reference to identify how the symptoms are interfering with daily life. Clients can also identify what they do for themselves to help relieve their symptoms. This maintains a client's position as a whole person capable of taking responsibility for and participating in the healing process.

AGGRAVATING

Aggravating circumstances should be specific to home, work and play. Sitting or standing for long periods of time commonly causes an increase in symptoms. If this is the case, find out how long the client can sit or stand before the symptom begins or worsens, and relate that to activities done normally before the injury. For example:

> Increased pain with prolonged sitting or standing. Changes positions every 15 minutes to avoid pain. Sits at computer for job, reads for recreation, stands often in kitchen for home chores.

Aggravating circumstances may also be listed as activities the client can no longer do, or can no longer do without pain. For example:

> Unable to lift heavy objects over 25 pounds—job requires lifting, workouts include Nautilus, small children at home require lifting. Unable to drive without pain—35 mile commute to work, picks children up from day care, has planned a driving vacation through the Canyon Lands next week. Currently must stop reading after 20 minutes, housework after 10 minutes.

When daily activities change dramatically but symptoms remain constant, a look at aggravating circumstances may reveal progress that might otherwise go undetected. Often, when clients are recovering from traumatic injuries, the better they feel, the more they attempt to do. They are eager to return to work, to get back to their hobbies and activities. As a result, there is no improvement in symptoms; the symptoms may even worsen. Rather than assuming that there is no progress, document the changes in activities. This will explain the lack of progress with the symptoms and prove progress regarding activities of daily living.

The Oswestry / Vernon/Mior Pain Questionnaire is an excellent way to document subjective information regarding loss of daily activities. Clients can fill this out prior to the session to avoid excessive time spent interviewing. It should be completed for the initial session, and then periodically as a part of status reports.

Clients may be advised by their attorney to keep a diary of their pain and its effect on their daily lives. This chart could serve that purpose; it can be photocopied and filled out by the client at home on a regular basis. Weekly or bi-monthly is considered to be timely.

Use the space on the SOAP chart for more personalized information than the Oswestry / Vernon/Mior allows. The client may have previously run marathons, rebuilt cars as a hobby or played an instrument in a local band. This detail tells much more of the effect of the symptoms on their lives than the questionnaire can. The Oswestry / Vernon/Mior, on the other hand, covers much more ground than you may think of doing or have time to do. Use both.

RELIEVING

Relieving circumstances include activities or treatments the client has found that alleviate the symptoms. Changing positions might help, as might taking frequent breaks. Stretching exercises, self massage or hydrotherapy techniques that the practitioner or other caregivers have suggested as homework may be beneficial. Particular massage techniques that have worked to relieve symptoms should be noted here. Clients often come back the following session and report what worked to relieve their symptoms.

Identifying aggravating and relieving circumstances helps the client to choose activities that promote health rather than those that create problems. It raises client consciousness and participation, and opens up the conversation between practitioner and client about supporting the treatments through awareness and change of the client's environment.

TIMING

The process of inquiry into current symptoms or client concerns will move much more smoothly if you follow a consistent format. Use of a detailed SOAP form will help insure completeness and consistency. See the Appendix for an entire sample case study.

If writing or spelling is an issue for you, recording information on a Dictaphone may ease the stress. Hiring a transcriber is cheaper than you may think, and is an easy alternative to scribbling notes. Transferring the taped information to a computer program may also speed up the process (and save a tree).

Subjective information may be documented during the interview process itself. While the client is undressing and getting on the table, the practitioner may complete this section of the chart.

CONCLUSION

Subjective data is reliable information, and valuable feedback from the client. It is useful for establishing treatment goals, documenting significant injury, proving progress, identifying the individual needs of the client and promoting client participation and freedom of choice. SOAP charting has a substantial capacity for recording client goals, symptoms, onset, and aggravating and relieving activities, all of which contribute to the necessary uses of subjective data.

Subjective information from example SOAP chart.

See Appendix 2 for complete form, page 71

S	**CLIENT GOALS / UPDATE**
	↓ ⓟ ↓ spasms ↑ rest
	LOCATION / SYMPTOMS / INTENSITY / FREQUENCY / DURATION / ONSET
	HA ⓟ S cons. post DOI - MVA
	neck ⓟ, M " " " "
	stiffness
	jaw ⓟ M interm. " " "
	ⓟ preventing restful sleep
	AGGRAVATING / RELIEVING CIRCUMSTANCES REGARDING ACTIVITIES OF DAILY LIVING
	A: driving, sitting, standing, reading, lifting, exercise, housework, childcare
	R: ice, advil, chiro. adj.

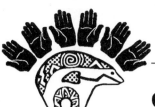

Chapter 3: *Objective Information*

Objective information includes your findings regarding the client's health: visual and palpable observations, test results, treatment goals, and massage techniques. In the past, insurance companies gave more weight to objective than to subjective information due to the greater credibility of the unbiased expert. More and more, of late, they are considering the client's (subjective) information to be as important.

It remains imperative to document only what is within your scope of practice. Be consistent and clear in your documentation. Stick to what you can clearly and confidently defend in court. Use what you are tested on in your state boards as guidelines: if you are expected to know it for the examination, you may use it in your practice. Standardize information gathering and document your findings uniformly. This will help create credibility for you and for your profession.

VISUAL OBSERVATIONS

Visual observations effectively document compromises in joint integrity, irregularities in movement patterns, breathing inconsistencies, and obvious deformities. These observations are quick to make and to note, and are equally quickly re-evaluated at any point in the massage. This provides constant feedback on the effectiveness of the treatment choices.

Visual observations include postural analysis, limps, muscle guarding or holding patterns, inconsistencies in movement, atrophy, hypertrophy, bruises, abrasions, scars, swelling, redness or pallor, skin irregularities, varicose veins, and breathing patterns. Many of the visual observations may be noted by drawing on the human figures on the SOAP charts, as shown here.

Postural analysis from example SOAP chart.

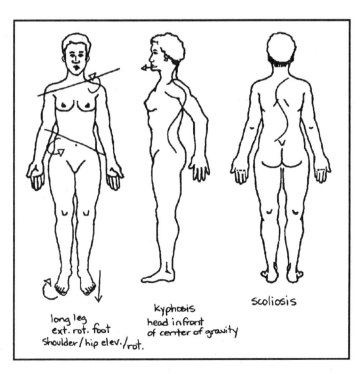

long leg
ext. rot. foot
shoulder / hip elev. / rot.

kyphosis
head in front
of center of gravity

scoliosis

Adding to the key will allow others to make sense of your additional unique drawings. Posture is easily noted on the forms by drawing skewed lines to depict elevations and arrows for rotations. Other information, such as breathing descriptions, may be more easily noted in the space provided for written information.

Many signs of shock can be visually noted, like skin pallor, sweaty goose flesh, and uneven dilation of the pupils, as well as rapid shallow breathing. People experiencing chronic pain may have such disruption in their nervous systems that they are often in a mild state of shock. Note this and treat accordingly.

Some visual observations are obvious, for example, prosthetics and paralysis. They are often omitted because they seem so blatant. It is important to sketch them on your SOAP chart even if they are written in the medical history; often they are the key to determining a relationship with the compensational dysfunctions in other parts of the body. Noting them will help you keep the big picture in mind.

Observe clients closely. Watch how they walk, sit, and turn to look behind themselves. Look for losses of function that result in compensational movements, or staggered movements that have lost their smooth flow. People may turn their bodies instead of their heads when looking over their shoulders. Observe uneven movements, like one arm that swings wildly while the other is held tightly to the side.

Some practitioners watch the eyes for irregular patterns of movement to assess dysfunctions in other body parts, and, as treatment progresses, will recheck the eye movement for smoothness to determine effectiveness of treatment.

Irregular movement patterns are a valuable visual observation. These are best seen during range of motion (ROM) active testing or when the client is least aware of being observed and is moving "normally". Patterns can easily be noted by watching your client enter the room, sit, stand up from a chair, walk down the hallway, turn to speak, or look over a shoulder, all without formal scrutiny. The more natural the movement, the more effective the testing situation. Breathing or walking done under scrutiny is rarely natural.

Postural analysis is an integral part of visual observations. If it's done in front of a mirror, or with photographs as is common with Rolfers, the client can see what you point out to be important. Clients relate to tangible visible information. The changes in posture as a result of the massage are also easily demonstrated, and the client can see the efficacy of massage as a therapy.

Assessing the posture of the client can locate the problematic holding patterns that are commonly the result of old, poorly healed injuries, or the result of repetitive uneven movements. Compensational holding patterns are usually more troublesome in the long run than the initial injury. An imbalance in the pelvis, for example, may result in uneven shoulder height. This causes the head to be held tightly on one side which may result in an impinged nerve and cause pain or numbness in the hand. A well-balanced massage session addresses all holding patterns as well as the key problem areas.

The common areas for observing posture are at the ears, the shoulders, the scapulae, the hips, the knees and the feet. The figure on the SOAP chart has lines drawn to facilitate comparisons. Height differences or elevations are observed, as well as rotations, inversions, eversions, leg length variances, and joint compromises. If a joint cannot be fully extended with relaxed muscles in a neutral position, it is considered to be compromised. Scoliosis, kyphosis, and lordosis are a few of the spinal dysfunctions easily noted on the figures.

Muscle tightness or spasms compromise the integrity of a joint. This may result in many of these postural adaptations. Occasionally bone deformity or disease, rather than soft tissue, causes the posture problem. A diagnosis from a primary caregiver can determine that. The intention of postural assessment is not to determine the cause or diagnose the injury, but to give the practitioner a foundation to compare progress to.

Breathing is an important visual observation. Breathing, like movement, is significant both as a way of assessing dysfunction and as a means of noting progress. As evidence of dysfunction, we note irregularities such as shallow, rapid, weak, uneven, or inconsistent patterns in breathing. Breathing is also a valuable way of checking the effectiveness of the treatment choices we are making. A goal of treatment is to restore breathing to a relaxed rate during the course of a massage session. As the breath deepens, one may assume progress on some level.

Attention to breath reminds clients of its importance and reinforces breath work as homework. Document pre- and post-massage breathing rates, but, more importantly, bring them to the attention of the clients. Introduce to their consciousness the sensation of relaxed breathing. Encourage them to practice relaxed breathing during stressful situations, and remind them that they have the power to return to this relaxed state at any time through deep breathing. Educating the client is very important.

Explain to your client that shallow breathing is a response to perceived danger. Millenia ago, we hypothesize, humans developed a "fight-or-flight" mechanism. Today the body responds to stress just as it once responded to life-threatening danger: in stressful situations, the body attempts to become small and still, so as not to be detected by its enemy. In the process, breathing is inhibited. When breathing remains shallow for an extended period of time, the muscles become contracted and muscle memory sets in. It becomes difficult to breathe deeply even when no stress or danger exists. Understanding the body's flight-or-fight mechanism regarding breathing can help bring understanding and patience to a frustrated client who feels no control of, or no awareness of, his breathing.

PALPABLE OBSERVATIONS

Palpable observations include any inconsistencies that can be felt in the soft tissue or joints. Massage practitioners have superior palpation skills, often more developed than the primary caregiver's. Therefore, this detailed information is a valuable resource for all caregivers involved. Some caregivers will use information from your notes to aid in writing their own reports. This creates a working environment that benefits you both.

Palpable observations may include tight muscles or hypertonicities, hypotonicities, spasms, trigger points, accupressure points, or any number of technical names for tender points, adhesions, scar tissue, swelling, congestion, temperature, pulses, rhythms, and so on.

Palpable observations are easily documented, and can be used to note progress. The use of human figures on the SOAP chart simplifies notation. Anything too complicated to draw on the figures can be written out in the space provided under visual/palpable observations.

Palpable observations as noted on the SOAP chart figures.

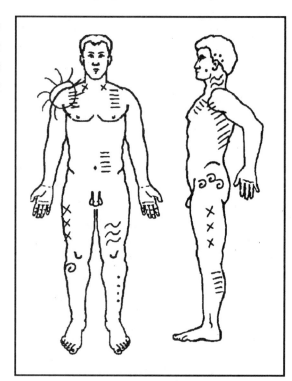

When documenting hypertonicities, one may choose to name the muscles individually in the space provided, to avoid confusion on the figures. Often there are so many hypertonicities that drawing them all on the figures would hide the other symbols. It is beneficial to rate the intensity of the hypertonicity as *mild,* Light *moderate* or *severe.* That is difficult to do on the figures, but not impossible. The space provided allows ample room to document each tight muscle and rate its intensity.

Documentation of these palpable findings includes identifying their specific location, the location of the referred pain site, and rating the intensity of the dysfunction for purposes of noting progress. For example: Trigger point right medial scalene, moderate pain to back of head. (Abbreviated: TP Ⓡ med. scal. M Ⓟ ➜ post head.)

TERMINOLOGY FOR PALPATION FINDINGS

Consistency in terminology and a clear understanding of what is being palpated is often a dilemma in our profession. We have Jones points, stress points, trigger points, accupressure points, etc...all varying interpretations or descriptions of similar phenomena. We can discuss the basics in this book and continue to leave the fine tuning open for interpretation according to specialty.

A question students frequently ask is, "What is the difference between hypertonicities and spasms?" The definition that works for me is that both are involuntary contractions of a muscle for any length of time, but that a spasm is painful before you touch it. A spasm is a protective response in the body that results in pain to prevent movement that may further the injury. A hypertonic muscle may or may not be painful with digital pressure.

Hypertonicities, spasms, tender points, trigger points and adhesions are some primary categories for palpation. Let's begin with a working definition of each.

Hypertonicity: An involuntarily tight or contracted muscle. May or may not be painful with digital pressure. May involve any part of or the whole of a muscle.

Spasm: An involuntary contraction of a muscle as a protective response to an injury or trauma, either emotional or physical. Is painful even without digital pressure.

Tender Point: Local, palpable, point specific, pain with digital pressure. May be a result of a micro-tear in the soft tissue, or of dysfunction in the proprioception of the soft tissue, or of a blockage of the energy flow of the area.

Trigger Point: Local, palpable, point specific, pain with digital pressure that refers pain to a specific location or area in the body seemingly unrelated to the tender point. A micro-tear in the soft tissue that has healed poorly and resulted in an over-stimulation of the proprioception in the muscle, setting up a pain-spasm-pain cycle in the nervous system. (Dr. J. Travell, *Myofascial Pain and Dysfunction)*

Adhesion: Scar tissue or collagen fibers that have bound muscle fibers to muscle fibers, muscles to muscles, connective tissue to muscles, connective tissue to bone and muscles to bone. A fascial restriction.

Primary caregivers, especially those in the western medical field, prefer the use of documented medical terminology. "Hypertonicity" carries more weight than "tight muscle", "adhesion" more than "knot". Trigger Points are very popular since the research of medical doctors Travell and Simmons. Any terms used to identify findings specific to technique specialties are acceptable, as long as you can discuss them fluently.

TEST RESULTS

Test results primarily refers to ROM (Range Of Motion) testing. Depending on your training it may also include muscle testing, Touch for Health, vertebral artery tests, Lasques Tests for sciatica or any other standardized testing format. All test results are objective information and are more substantial and less subjective than the visual or palpable observations. In other words, in situations involving insurance companies, the more test results within our scope of practice that substantiate significant injury, the more persuasive the case.

The use of those common standardized medical tests also aids in validating massage therapy. ROM testing is one of the best avenues for this purpose.

ROM TESTING

Range of motion testing is a valuable assessment tool in many health care professions. ROM test results substantiate significant injury, determine levels of severity of sprains and strains, identify stages of inflammation, and prove progress. It is one of the few assessment tools within the scope of practice of licensed massage practitioners, under the guise of Swedish gymnastics.

Every client can understand and relate to a decrease or increase in mobility and how that affects their lives. It can be very frustrating when one's ability to move and perform normal activities becomes restricted. Assessing ROM test results before treatment substantiates the limitations for the client. Re-testing ROM after massage sessions demonstrates the effectiveness of the treatment and proves progress as a result of the session. Periodic testing pre- and post-treatment shows continued progress, and gives the client evidence that the treatment is working. This proves to them that massage not only makes one feel better but is also a curative health care modality.

For the practitioner, one purpose of ROM testing is to aid in identifying problems and in assessing their severity in order to treat them safely, effectively and efficiently. Gathering empirical evidence is another purpose. In addition, the testing procedure helps assure the client of the practitioner's professionalism and trustworthiness. Testing will be the clients' first exposure to the practitioner's hands-on skills, and will influence their expectations of the actual massage, when they will be in a more vulnerable position.

The therapist identifies the pain-free or fully functional side of the body through the client's active test results, and continues to test the pain-free functional side of the body first through the remainder of the active and all of the passive and resistive movements. Handling the pain-free side confidently and safely aids in establishing trust and minimizes muscle guarding when testing the painful dysfunctional side. It also provides a set of "normal" measurements for comparison and for assessing dysfunction.

Determining the "end feel" of active and passive movement is one of three assessment goals of ROM testing. Identifying pain and its location is the second assessment goal. Assessing the strength of muscles during resistive ROM is the third. When testing, assure clients that if the pain causes too much discomfort to continue the movement, they may stop. Often, however, the pain is not disabling and sometimes disappears as the movement continues. The key thing to remember is that the end feel is usually where the discomfort is found and those end feels should only be held for a second for identification purposes. It is more important to identify and document the problem than to avoid a second or two of discomfort. Pain that limits the ability to reach the end range is valuable information and requires documentation.

The location of pain may identify the specific area of the dysfunction. The pain or discomfort may be in the muscle stretch itself, signifying a hypertonicity. The pain may be found on the right upper cervical region with both right and left rotation, demonstrating a ligament or joint problem. Locating the pain during testing also directs the practitioner to concentrate treatment to that area, isolating the problem areas for fast efficient treatment.

The pattern of the movement is equally important to note. Some movements may seem jagged or staggered. This indicates a need to reset the proprioceptors in the muscles to obtain smooth movement.

A practitioner must always be aware of compensational movement patterns and give clear instructions to provide a neutral testing environment in order to get accurate test results. The body naturally adapts to weak areas through changing movement patterns for protection against further injury. Not all compensations can be prevented. Noting compensational patterns also aids in identifying dysfunctions.

DOCUMENTATION OF ROM TESTING

It is necessary, in documenting test results, to establish normal ROM for each individual. Pre-injury status is difficult to determine, of course, if testing was not done immediately prior to an injury. Other factors, too, may affect what is considered normal. Normal for a dancer varies drastically from what is normal for a non-athlete. When a dysfunction is one-sided, the opposite side may be used for a normal comparison. Otherwise client feedback is required to determine what is normal for them.

Be sure to specify right, left or bilateral when referring to joints.

Documenting ROM testing includes:

1. Identifying:
    a. right, left, or bilateral
    b. muscle or joint
    c. action or muscle being stretched
    d. hyper- or hypo-mobility
    e. presence and location of pain

2. Qualifying:
    a. intensity of hypo- or hyper-mobility
    b. intensity of pain
    c. strength or lack thereof

ROM testing is done to determine an increase or a decrease from normal ROM. Arrows may be used to denote hyper- or hypo-mobility. Normal ROM may be referred to as WNL—within normal limits. Pain is either present and can be noted through a qualifying term, or is nonexistent, in which case you use a symbol for no pain.

Qualifying the intensity of the pain or the increase or decrease in mobility provides a mode of comparison for proving progress. Due to the nature of soft tissue repair, 100% mobility may never be achieved. Rather than simply showing a decrease in ROM session after session, demonstrate the change from a moderate limitation in movement to a mild limitation.

Degrees of angles are commonly used to qualify mobility. For example, normal active cervical lateral flexion is 45 degrees bilaterally. As massage therapists, we must use caution when documenting degrees without proper tools or training. If an injury case is reviewed in court and the chiropractor, physical therapist, and massage practitioner all have ROM testing showing different degrees for the same actions, who will they believe?

Probably not us, since we lack medical training. Attorneys commonly advise all health care professionals to avoid the use of percentages and degrees to qualify subjective test results and client progress because of possible discrepancies. To avoid any conflict, use a simple three point scale.

LIGHT

Mild, moderate and *severe* are effective adjectives for massage therapists to use to qualify levels of severity of a dysfunction. Hypermobility, hypomobility and pain can all be effectively qualified through these adjectives. When a three point scale is too limiting a plus or a minus may be added to each, creating a nine point scale of evaluation. This allows for comparison without room for invalidation.

Example of ROM documentation of client's neck .

NECK												
FLEXION *	↓M		M		↓M		M		↓M		M	
EXTENSION *	too much mm guarding				too Øful to test				↓M		M	
LATERAL FLEXION	↓M	↓M	M	M	↓M	↓M	M	M	WNL	WNL	☺	☺
ROTATION	↓L	↓L	L	L	↓M	↓M	M	M	WNL	WNL	☺	☺

See Appendix 2 for complete form, page 72

TREATMENT GOALS

Treatment goals are an important part of objective information. They define the intention of the massage choices and demonstrate the curative value of massage. They insure that your treatment plan has a purpose. Make them as specific as possible. Draw from your client's goals, and from your subjective and objective findings.

The most important place to derive the treatment goals from is your clients. Clients' concerns for the day may or may not have anything to do with their symptoms or with your observations and test results. It is important to maintain perspective on your personal agenda with your clients, on what you think you can accomplish with them, and on their desires. Often these are not the same. Remember that you can only take clients as far as they are willing to go in their relationship with their bodies. If a person is not ready to let go of poor posture, for example, then all of your efforts will be in vain.

If your client is eager to rid her body of symptoms, then focus your treatment goals on her symptoms, your visual and palpable observations, and test results. You may not have time to actually address all the goals in the treatment time allotted, so prioritize them. Use your status reports to identify all of your goals, and then choose appropriate ones on a daily basis.

Be realistic about your expectations, and always go for the fifty percent release rather than a hundred percent. It is not necessary to fix a problem instantly or to get rid of a symptom totally. Healing takes time, and over-treatment is an easy trap to fall into. Keep the entire body in mind and don't get caught up in "fixing" a single area. Move around; attempt to get releases in one area through working another. Work with systems instead of spots.

In charting these goals, you might use abbreviations like:

↓ ⑨—*decrease pain*
↑ ROM—*increase range of motion*
↓ adh.—*decrease adhesions*
↑ resp.—*increase respiration*
↓ sh. elev.—*decrease shoulder elevation*

Chose specific treatment modalities or techniques to accomplish your goals. This gives your treatment structure and direction. Be flexible about adjusting your goals or your treatment choices. If you are not achieving the desired results, try another technique. Stay in close communication with your client. Ask if the symptoms are getting better or worse with the treatment. If the symptoms worsen, try another technique. Beware of over-treating. Signs of over-treatment include an increase in the symptoms, increased signs of inflammation, goose-flesh, nausea, and muscle guarding. It is very easy to over-treat.

MASSAGE

The massage portion of the chart documents the type of massage provided in the session and the order in which it was given. This is helpful for several reasons.

The first is that clients may return and request the same treatment as before. Since it was effective, they want the exact same thing again. You should be able to reproduce your session reasonably well from your notes.

Secondly, you want to be able to refer back to your notes and see what treatment techniques were effective in accomplishing the results recorded. By referring to the body part listed and seeing what techniques were used you should be able to infer what was successful for that particular person.

Thirdly, if an insurance company is reading the notes, or you are called upon to testify, you must be able to defend your treatment choices. Exactly what you did and why should be recorded in your chart notes.

Document your massage in two ways. First give a big picture of the massage, include all the body parts touched, the order, and the general sense of the flow, style and pace. Include the foundation of your technique, like Swedish massage, Cranio-sacral therapy or Shiatsu. Then give details regarding the particular techniques used to treat specific findings and accomplish each of the individual goals set. You needn't write down everything you do; just give the highlights. For example:

> Full body Swedish massage. Prone: Back—linear friction—erector spinae, crossfiber friction—levator scapula. Hips—direct pressure—piriformis trigger point. Legs—compression. Supine: Neck—muscle energy technique lateral flexion bilateral. Arms—shoulder jostling. Legs—crossfiber friction—illiotibial band. Feet—reflexology.

Or, abbreviated:

FB SW Ⓜ
Prone: Back—lin. fric.—erec. sp.
       XFF—lev. scap.
       Hips—DP—piri. TP
       Legs—comp.
Supine: Neck—MET lat. flex. BL
       Arms—sh. jost.
       Legs—XFF ITB
       Feet—reflex.

TIMING OF DOCUMENTATION

Much objective information may be documented on the SOAP chart before the hands-on part of the session actually begins. The exceptions are the palpable observations and the massage portion. Postural assessment and test results may be documented in the treatment room with the client before the session. Treatment goals can be discussed and decided upon, and a plan for the session can be determined.

Wait to document the massage until after the session is over. This allows for flexibility. You may find that your agenda for the massage was not effective and you needed to change your plans mid-stream. You may also have modified your treatment goals. Simply cross out any unnecessary information and add what is pertinent.

When you exit the room after the session, immediately draw on the figures provided, while the image of the body is still fresh in your mind. Draw the palpable findings such as hypertonicities, adhesions, and trigger points. If you have a tendency to forget easily, take mini time-outs to jot down bits of information as you go. Clients will understand the breaks in contact if you inform them of what you are doing and its importance to their care.

Documenting in this manner is a great time-saver. Use the time during your interview, the time while the client is undressing, and the time they are dressing after the massage to write on the chart. During the closing interview, discuss and record your assessment and your plan. You will find that almost the entire charting procedure can be done during the time spent with the client. There is no need to stay after work or take breaks between clients to chart. Your time is valuable; charting time should be part of each session.

SUMMARY

In the objective portion, document things you observe, feel, and discover to be true, set goals and determine how to accomplish them. This information will identify problem areas, substantiate symptoms, prove significant injury and describe the massage session.

Objective information from example SOAP chart.

See Appendix 2 for complete form, page 71

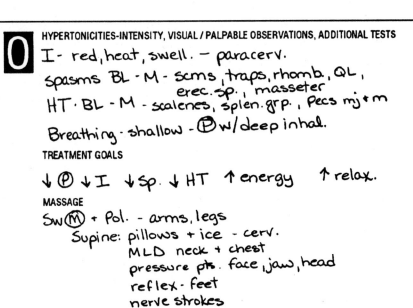

O HYPERTONICITIES-INTENSITY, VISUAL / PALPABLE OBSERVATIONS, ADDITIONAL TESTS

I - red, heat, swell. — paracerv.
Spasms BL - M - scms, traps, rhomb., QL,
      erec. sp., masseter
HT · BL - M - scalenes, splen. grp., Pecs mj + m

Breathing - shallow - Ⓟ w/ deep inhal.

TREATMENT GOALS

↓Ⓟ ↓I ↓Sp. ↓HT ↑energy   ↑relax.

MASSAGE

Sw Ⓜ + Pol. - arms, legs
   Supine: pillows + ice - cerv.
           MLD neck + chest
           pressure pts. face, jaw, head
           reflex - feet
           nerve strokes

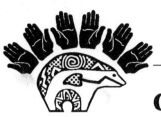

Chapter 4: *Assessment*

This is the one section where the standard SOAP chart must be modified for our use. Since massage therapists are unable to diagnose, the diagnosis/prognosis portion of assessment is replaced by changes that are an immediate result of the massage session.

Under assessment you record the changes in the client's symptoms, musculo-skeletal system, function or mobility, posture and so on, that are an immediate result of the treatment. Monitor these changes throughout the massage, and be sure to re-test ROM and posture at the end of the session. Assessment is used to determine or reinforce the effectiveness of specific treatment techniques, as well as to note the progress of the client. Change may be qualified by rating the change in the levels of severity of the symptoms.

Labor and Industries requires massage practitioners to prove progress before granting a continuation of treatment. Other insurance companies require proof that this is "reasonable and necessary care" to justify coverage, as none will pay for merely palliative services. This is easily proven through the documentation of subjective and objective changes as a result of treatment. Re-testing and re-evaluating throughout the massage sessions and the course of treatments will show this progress.

All treatment goals should be addressed in this section, and tests appropriate to treatment given should be re-administered. Posture, ROM and others are easily done post-massage. Changes in symptoms should be noted. Hypertonicities, adhesions, inflammation and trigger points can all be assessed during the massage. Changes that could be taken for granted can be included. An increase in circulation or in lymphatic flow, an ease in breathing, and parasympathetic responses are a few changes that are considered physiological responses to Swedish massage and may also be mentioned.

Qualify the amount of change you see and feel. Demonstrate the effectiveness of the treatment choices in accomplishing these changes. Was there a mild, moderate or significant increase in cervical rotation? Was it a mild, moderate or significant decrease in hypertonicities? Wherever the intensity of a symptom or finding is noted, the change should be qualified. For example:

> Mild increase in left cervical flexion, change in hypertonicity of the right levator scapula from moderate to mild.

Abbreviated:

> L ↑ Ⓛ cerv. lat. flex., Ⓡ lev. scap. ↓ HT M → L

Perhaps a technique caused a symptom to worsen rather than improve, or caused no change in the symptom at all. That is appropriate to note also. For example:

No change in headache pain. (Abbreviated: △ HA Ⓟ)

Not all goals may have been addressed in the session. Time may not have permitted it. In that case, cross out the goal from the section above. That will demonstrate a desire to obtain the goal, but no time to try. If you simply wrote "no change", one might assume that the treatment was ineffective. Be as explicit as possible whenever possible.

Use as many descriptive words as possible. Be specific in your use of terminology. It is difficult to quantify a change in relaxation, or to sound professional when you say, "The knot melted". Use terms consistent with your objective data and speak to your most technical audience.

Assessment is the means by which progress is proven. Documenting this change demonstrates the curative powers of massage to the client, to the referring caregivers and to the insurance companies. Thoroughness of charting in this section will encourage widespread use of massage for preventive health care and for the treatment of soft tissue injuries.

TIMING

Treatment, assessment and plan can be recorded while clients are dressing, and discussed with them before they leave.

Remember, assessment is the most valuable section on the SOAP chart. It is usually what gets you paid, and what keeps referrals coming. It is the proof that *Hands Heal*.

Assessment information from example SOAP chart.

See Appendix 2 for complete form, page 71

A	CHANGES DUE TO MASSAGE

↓ I - M △
↓ HT - L △ overall   ↑ Rom lat flex L△
↓ Sp - L△ neck   △̸ LB M △ jaw
↓ Ⓟ M → L⁺ neck △̸ LB M → L⁻ jaw
↓ HA S → M
↑ bal / relax overall

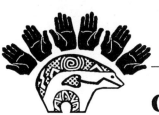

Chapter 5: *Plan*

Plan is the portion of the chart in which to suggest a treatment frequency and a focus for future massage sessions, to encourage client participation in between sessions, and to set both long term and short term goals. It includes the following categories: treatment plan, massage frequency, and homework.

TREATMENT PLAN

Your treatment plan will take into account what worked, what didn't work, what you didn't have time to address, and what you want to make sure you work on next time. It should recognize the clients' individual needs and preferences, the things that make them feel safer, more relaxed, what they might like to begin or end a session with, the techniques or positions they prefer. For example:

Begin with feet, treat neck side lying.

Abbreviated:

1st feet, neck—SL

Note any specific techniques that worked well to accomplish specific goals; you may want to use them again. Include your clients' feedback on what they found to be especially beneficial, what they would prefer to leave out or to include in the next session. For example:

Continue myofascial release on left medial hamstring.

Abbreviated:

Cont. MFR Ⓛ Med. Ham.

You might also note what techniques were not effective. For example, if you attempted cross-fiber friction and the client had an adverse reaction, you could note that and set a time when it might be worth trying the technique again. (Abbreviated: ⓍⒻ → I ↑, re-eval 3 wks.)

Or you might, five minutes before the end of a session, find a possible relationship between a specific muscle and the client's symptom. There is no time to address the discovery that session, so you note it in this section of the SOAP chart and plan to build your next session around it. For example:

Check psoas. (Abbreviated: ✔ psoas)

If no change has been noted under assessment you may have ideas regarding other possible approaches. This may also be noted under plan. Often, as soon as you walk out of the session you have an inspiration about a possible treatment technique. Don't risk forgetting it; write it down under Plan.

For the sake of efficiency, you might want to fill out the Plan portion of the chart immediately after the session, either while the client is dressing or during the closing interview.

MASSAGE FREQUENCY

Massage frequency is a projected number of massage sessions over a set period of time. Designate an end to a series of massages to allow for goal setting and an opportunity to re-evaluate the intent and focus of the sessions. (This is when you will write status reports.) Agreeing to once a week for four weeks increases the chance that the client will stick it out for four weeks to allow progress to become apparent. It also gives the client an out if the treatments are not working satisfactorily. And it provides an avenue to discuss other alternatives, and encourages a team approach.

Suggest a length of time for consecutive sessions. Discuss with your clients how many sessions it may take to reach a desired goal. Emphasize that what took ten years of stress to develop cannot be corrected in one massage; the body will not change that quickly. It will require a well-rounded approach to healing, including regular massage, exercise, and a change in the environment that created the dysfunction, or at least a change in how the client responds to the environment.

This is all done through Plan. Promote long term and short term goal setting to assist in this approach to healing. Use your (status report sessions) to help determine appropriate goals. Schedule in the status reports to insure proper evaluation and time for discussion of the plan. You might decide, for example, on twelve sessions, with one status report session at the sixth session and one at the twelfth.

When the pre-determined number of massages has been completed, re-evaluation can take place. Until then encourage the client to stick it out. This may require making minor adjustments; results do not always occur as quickly as one may anticipate. Re-evaluation may discover a need to change the approach or the frequency of treatment. You may decide to reduce or increase the number of sessions. Massage has a cumulative effect, and after a while one may receive the same results with sessions every other week as one initially did with weekly sessions.

When documenting the massage frequency, state the frequency, the time line, and the re-evaluation date. For example: 1x / wk / 4 wks / 10-3-92. If the frequency is prescribed by the primary care giver, add "as prescribed" to your statement. You may choose to omit it from the SOAP chart; it will be documented in the referring prescription.

HOMEWORK

Homework is based on the idea of client responsibility and participation in the healing process. Often life changes are required to gain health or to maintain a desired function in daily living. Actively participating in the process, like actively choosing the treatment modalities, increases the likelihood of success of the treatment. Due to the nature of soft tissue injury repair, clients must often make lifestyle changes to regain maximum function. Stretching and strengthening must become habit, a part of everyday living.

As the frequency of treatments decreases and the amount of self care increases, a sense of well-being and power replaces any sense of being a victim that the client may have had. People who suffer from injuries resulting from the carelessness of others often feel victimized. This can perpetuate a "fix me" attitude. Including the client in the treatment planning, and the gentle introduction of homework can thwart this unhealthy attitude. Active participation on behalf of the client reduces the number of re-injuries or exacerbations of the old injury and keeps people working and functioning more fully in their lives.

Homework must be tailored to meet the personality and needs of each client. It should fit into the client's lifestyle, it should be goal-oriented, and each exercise should build on the last. Set the client up for success. Be realistic in the goal setting. If, for example, the client's goal is to run competitively again, homework might begin with walking 20 minutes a day for the first 2 weeks, then increasing the time to 40 minutes a day, and later to 60 minutes, then starting to jog a mile a day...2 miles a day...and so on.

Clients' lifestyles vary considerably. Some people have never been active in their lives, and need very specific instructions. Others may be jocks, and know more exercises than you do. Some people may be more concerned with doing it right, or how much time it takes. For just about everyone the challenge is in how they can incorporate it into their already busy lives.

Success with homework has a lot to do with how you present it. Homework should be something that clients can relate to on an emotional level, where they feel or sense the benefits. It is important to fit a program to each individual's style, so that it's simple enough to remember, not so overwhelming that they give up, and short enough that they can fit it into their spare time. This can be accomplished with patience over a period of time as you get to know each other.

Give one exercise at a time. Increase homework gradually as clients reach their goals. If one exercise can be done successfully every day for one or two weeks, add one more exercise. This will help them create time in their lives and will develop the habit of self care. "They" say it takes 27 days to make a habit. Doing any self care daily, no matter how small, will set clients up for a lifetime pattern of self care.

Long, complicated exercises are less apt to be successful due to the myriad of possible problems. "As soon as I got home I forgot everything you said." Even writing instructions down can be fruitless. "I lost the piece of paper." "The dog ate it." "The diagram you drew didn't make any sense the next day." "I had time over the weekend but as soon as I got back to work I had too much else to do."

Homework can include trying alternatives to pain pills. Suggest, for example, that clients try an ice pack instead of aspirin for pain. These don't have to be used on a routine basis, three times a day, but simply whenever one is experiencing discomfort. Support pillows are another alternative to pain pills. Suggest pillows in their chairs at work, in the car, at home in bed. Cervical pillows and lumbar support pillows can decrease pain tremendously and give people a sense of power in participating in promoting better health.

Make sure your suggestions don't conflict with instructions from a primary caregiver, however. Meet with them to inform them of any opinions you have; use the team approach with them as well as with your clients. Most caregivers are open to suggestions that are presented appropriately.

Begin the homework process by helping your clients become aware of the activities which seem to cause them pain or which increase their tension. This will build body awareness of sensation, and mental awareness of what is triggering the dysfunction. You might have clients stop every hour at work and take ten deep breaths. During this time they may do a body scan and notice what their body feels like. Two weeks later you might add an eyes-closed affirmation to their ten deep breaths, for example, "I am relaxed and present in my body. I recognize what causes me tension and am actively working on relaxing during those situations." Two weeks later have them drink a glass of water every two hours.

Once body awareness is established and clients know they can participate in achieving better health without a large time commitment, add routines including hydrotherapy, stretching and strengthening. Motivation is necessary to encourage time commitments necessary for this level of participation. Short term and long term goal setting around these tasks can be helpful.

In goal setting it is important to keep a clear perspective on what's possible or achievable to prevent a sense of failure. Given the nature of soft tissue injuries, 100% recovery is not always a possibility. Educate your clients on the importance of daily participation to achieve full function. Long term goals may include running marathons, returning to normal work duty, or being pain free. When this is the case the emphasis needs to be on a series of short term goals. Short term goals may include one hour of pain-free activity, or returning to work half-time. Be flexible. One can always amend goals.

Short term goals are similar to and closely integrated with homework in that they need to reflect the client's lifestyle and need to be supported by the homework given. Homework is the means for accomplishing those goals.

Be as specific as possible when documenting homework. You need to be able to follow up on precisely what homework you gave, in order to be supportive.

TIMING

Short term goals should be set weekly and monthly, and long term goals set over three, six, nine and twelve month periods. Homework should be given weekly according to the progress being made. Goals should be reviewed regularly and modified when necessary. This actively engages the client, and creates a team-work approach to healing.

Planning section from example SOAP chart.

See Appendix 2 for complete form, page 71

SUGGESTED TREATMENT PLAN

2x wk / 4 wk - re·eval 5.13 per 'script.
P. Rom cerv. avail. next tx.

HOMEWORK

ice packs 2-3 x/dy neck or prn
↑ short rest periods

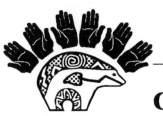

Chapter 6: *Status Reports*

Status reports are periodic summaries of a client's status. In them complete ROM testing, postural analysis, subjective and objective findings are documented. This allows for evaluation of the client's treatment, progress and goals. A detailed SOAP chart format is used, plus several additional forms. Progress can be summarized in segments, from status report to status report, or over the entire case history, from the first treatment to the present.

A status report is done at the initial visit to give a big picture of the client's physical status, and to note details that need not be repeated in the daily SOAP charts. A full body perspective is important in determining a plan for the first five to eight sessions. Status reports are then updated periodically to summarize progress, and to give the full body update to help plan the next series of treatments.

Regular status reports make the weekly massage sessions flow smoothly. They suggest goals for individual sessions. Specific details can be checked and re-checked in one session without having to test everything to determine the needs of the day.

In brief, status reports are useful for the following purposes:

- to set goals and to plan a series of massage treatments
- to summarize progress, both short term and long term
- to assess the effectiveness of treatments
- to update referring care givers (rather than sending them every SOAP chart)
- as an easy reference for review for the LMP
- as an easy reference for writing narrative reports

Status reports show how effective various treatments have been, as well as the pace of the client's healing process. With this information the client and the practitioner can discuss reasonable expectations for the future. Status reports are useful for setting goals and devising a plan for a series of massage treatments.

Status reports can also be used to refresh your memory before massage sessions. It is important to review a client's file immediately before treatment to recall specific information and prepare for the session. The status reports are useful summaries for this purpose. You could, for example, review an entire file by reading three or four status reports. This is far more efficient than reading twenty SOAP charts.

When writing narrative reports, the status reports again make easy reference material. You can use the relatively few status reports to compose your narratives rather than combing through many SOAP's of information.

Referring caregivers appreciate receiving these updates on your mutual client's status. SOAP charts are cumbersome for them to read. The status reports will summarize progress, demonstrate the treatment modalities used, and show projected plans for future treatments. Doctors are often very interested in your objective findings, as LMP's usually are the only ones with time to do regular thorough full body assessments.

WHAT DOES THE STATUS REPORT CONTAIN?

All information obtained for a SOAP chart should be obtained for a status report, only in greater detail. A description of all current symptoms should be included, not just the immediate concerns. This will save time in the interim sessions, allowing more time for the client's daily needs and goals rather than symptoms that have little to do with that day's concerns.

Status report forms are roomy, detailed SOAP charts. The SOAP forms used in this section are recommended for use on a regular basis when learning to use a SOAP format because of their detail. As you become more fluent in charting you may opt for a more simplified version of the SOAP chart. Variations on the charts are presented in this text to allow for personalization and freedom of expression.

SUBJECTIVE

There are several forms that can be used to summarize subjective information. Most of them require the client to fill them out. This is an important time-saving device. The more information you can gather before the session actually begins, the more time you will have for the massage.

I recommend using a form that has clients draw their current symptoms on human figures. This is what we refer to as the Personal Status Report. Often people find it easier to write or draw their symptoms than to talk about them. These forms use the same figures as the SOAP chart, but larger, and with a simplified set of symbols, for the clients' ease.

Example of Personal Status Report filled out by client.

See Appendix 2 for complete form, page 70

Name: Ms. Ideal Client   Date: 4·17·92

Identify CURRENT symptomatic areas in your body by drawing the symbols on the figures below.

KEY:
○ Circle areas of PAIN

X "X" over areas of JOINT AND MUSCLE STIFFNESS

⧙ Draw a squiggly lines along the areas of NUMBNESS OR TINGLING

╫ Mark SCARS, BRUISES or OPEN WOUNDS

The Oswestry/Vernon/Mior Pain Questionnaire is another form clients can fill out before their massage. This documents the symptoms' effects on the client's ability to function in daily life. It is specific to neck and back injuries, but other body parts may be referred to in order to meet individual needs.

Example of Oswestry/Vernon/ Mior Pain Question-naire filled out by client.

See Appendix 2 for complete form, page 69

NECK PAIN AND DISABILITY INDEX (Vernon-Mior)

Name: _Ms. Ideal Client_   Date: _4·17·92_

This questionnaire has been designed to give the health care provider information as to how your neck pain has affected your ability to manage everyday life. Please answer every section and mark in each section only the **ONE** box which applies to you. We realize you may consider that two of the statements in any one section relate to you, but please just mark the box which most closely describes your problem today.

SECTION 1- PAIN INTENSITY
- ☐ I have no pain at the moment.
- ☐ The pain is very mild at the moment.
- ☐ The pain is moderate at the moment.
- ☒ The pain is fairly severe at the moment.
- ☐ The pain is very severe at the moment.
- ☐ The pain is the worst imaginable at the moment.

SECTION 2- PERSONAL CARE (washing, dressing etc.)
- ☐ I can look after myself normally without causing pain.
- ☐ I can look after myself normally but it causes extra pain.
- ☒ It is painful to look after myself and I am slow and careful.
- ☐ I need some help but manage most of my personal care.
- ☐ I need help every day in most aspects of self care.
- ☐ I do not get dressed, I wash with difficulty and I stay in bed.

SECTION 3- LIFTING
- ☐ I can lift heavy weights without extra pain.
- ☐ I can lift heavy weights but it gives extra pain.
- ☐ Pain prevents me from lifting heavy weights off the floor, but I can manage if they are conveniently positioned, for example on a table.
- ☒ Pain prevents me from lifting heavy weights, but I can manage light to medium weights if they are conveniently positioned.
- ☐ I can lift very light weights.
- ☐ I cannot lift or carry anything at all.

SECTION 4- READING
- ☐ I can read as much as I want to with no pain in my neck.
- ☐ I can read as much as I want to with slight pain in my neck.
- ☐ I can read as much as I want to with moderate pain in my neck.
- ☐ I can't read as much as I want because of moderate pain in my neck.
- ☒ I can hardly read at all because of severe pain in my neck.
- ☐ I cannot read at all.

SECTION 6- CONCENTRATION
- ☐ I can concentrate fully when I want to with no difficulty.
- ☐ I can concentrate fully when I want to with slight difficulty.
- ☐ I have a fair degree of difficulty in concentrating when I want to.
- ☒ I have a great deal of difficulty in concentrating when I want to.
- ☐ I cannot concentrate at all.

SECTION 7- WORK
- ☐ I can do as much work as I want to.
- ☐ I can do my usual work but no more.
- ☐ I can do most of my usual work but no more.
- ☒ I cannot do my usual work.
- ☐ I can hardly do any work at all.
- ☐ I can't do any work at all.

SECTION 8- DRIVING
- ☐ I can drive my car without any neck pain.
- ☐ I can drive my car as long as I want with slight pain in my neck.
- ☐ I can drive my car as long as I want with moderate pain in my neck.
- ☐ I can't drive my car as long as I want because of moderate pain in my neck.
- ☒ I can hardly drive at all because of severe pain in my neck.
- ☐ I can't drive my car at all.

SECTION 9- SLEEPING
- ☐ I have no trouble sleeping.
- ☐ My sleep is slightly disturbed (less than one hour sleepless).
- ☐ My sleep is mildly disturbed (1-2 hrs. sleepless).
- ☒ My sleep is moderately disturbed (2-3 hrs. sleepless).
- ☐ My sleep is greatly disturbed (3-5 hrs. sleepless).
- ☐ My sleep is completely disturbed (5-7 hrs. sleepless).

SECTION 10- RECREATION.
- ☐ I am able to engage in all my recreation activities with no neck pain at all.

The Injury Information Form, completed for the initial visit, provides the details regarding the onset of the symptoms. This includes the biomechanics of the movement involved as well as any external mechanisms that may have affected the outcome of the injury. Details such as these are helpful in streamlining treatment and determining the focus of the massage sessions. This form does not need to be updated in subsequent status reports.

OBJECTIVE

Complete range-of-motion testing should be done at this time, as only partial testing is done week by week. For example, during a status report session, the complete cervical range of motion testing may be done, whereas during a standard session, only lateral flexion of the neck may be tested pre- and post-treatment.

More than one section of the body may be tested during a status report session, especially if the problem is a complicated dysfunction with compensational postural patterns in various locations. This provides valuable information, although it may be time-consuming. ROM test results give you the most valid and substantial evidence of progress, second only to improved function in daily living. This information is especially necessary when working in conjunction with insurance companies and with primary caregivers.

Complete monthly ROM testing is important in spotting areas that need treatment. This aids in setting goals and in designing the treatment protocol for the next month's massage sessions. You might, for example, find that rotation is the most severely limited action during a status report session. With this information, you can concentrate the next few sessions of treatment, assessment and homework on techniques that will improve that action.

Thorough postural assessment is a part of every status report. A quick standing frontal analysis or a simple analysis of the client's posture while lying on the table during the massage is often all that is taken during interim sessions. All aspects, however, are observed during a status report session. This includes anterior, side and posterior views and leg length testing.

Palpable observations, as well as other visual observations, are noted over the entire body for a status report. For interim SOAP charts these may be noted only for the areas of focus. It is important to get a periodic view of the whole picture to see the overall effectiveness of the treatments.

ASSESSMENT

Status report assessments summarize the progress over the period of time between status reports. Some of this information is subjective—what the client reports after they leave the sessions. Be clear and document that information in the appropriate section. Much of the information consists of your observation of which symptoms are measurably improving and which remain the same. Here you may assess the choice of treatment techniques to date. Are the goals you and your client set being reached? Is it time to adjust the old plan?

PLAN

Status reports plan the treatment for the next series of sessions. The assessment allows you to review the success of the treatment to date. Here you and your client can discuss and determine the general make-up of the next several massages.

TIMING

Timing of status reports is commonly every five to eight sessions. Because status report sessions involve more paperwork and testing, schedule an extra half hour with the client. Record the necessary information while the client is present so paperwork doesn't pile up on your desk. If you schedule the extra time, your clients will still enjoy a full hour massage, and will reap the benefits of a good overview of their status. It is also an opportunity to involve clients in making decisions about future treatments.

Much of the subjective information can be gathered without taking time from the massage session. Clients can fill these forms out before the session begins if instructed to come in early. The objective tests' results may be recorded during the testing itself. The awkward moments come when you are trying to document the palpable observations without breaking up the massage time too much. This can be done tactfully with clear communication and an environment that supports status report time.

CLIENT PARTICIPATION

Status reports give the client an opportunity to participate in making treatment choices. They also give the practitioner an opportunity to discuss what is working and what isn't. This reinforces the new trend in health care which gives power to the patient, and also aids in establishing the validity of massage as a viable treatment modality.

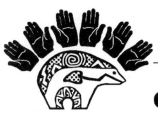

Chapter 7: *Narrative Reports*

Narrative reports summarize the client's case history to date. They are generally written either for lawyers, for use in personal injury cases, or for doctors, in order to update them on client progress. The content of the report will vary depending on its purpose.

Near the end of a personal injury case, a lawyer will often request a narrative report covering all treatment pertaining to the accident-related injuries in order to substantiate a client's claim. This will require a summary of the entire case history from start to finish. On average these reports will be four to six pages long—long enough for the information to support the client's case, but not so long as to be cumbersome.

On the other hand, reports written for primary care givers will be fairly short—just one or two pages. Many physicians prefer to receive these narrative summaries instead of copies of your chart notes in order to monitor their clients' progress with regard to your care. Sending them can be a good marketing device for you; physicians appreciate good record-keeping skills, and are apt to recommend you to other doctors if you demonstrate them. (Sending these short narratives to keep the referring care-givers updated is considered a courtesy, and you will not normally charge for them.)

WHAT BELONGS IN A NARRATIVE REPORT

Narratives follow a SOAP format. They include the client's initial subjective information, the practitioner's initial objective findings, what treatment techniques were used and why, suggested homework, assessment of changes as a result of treatment, and then the client's current subjective information, the practitioner's current objective findings, and the prognosis, if requested, including a suggested plan for continued treatments.

You begin a narrative report by describing the circumstances of the client's injury. Note the date that you first treated the client and the name of the referring primary caregiver. State all the initial presenting symptoms and any aggravating circumstances. List your test results, visual observations, and palpation findings. Now discuss the treatment techniques you used, where you used them, and why. Then present the changes that resulted from the treatment. This will give the reader a picture of the client's condition right after the accident, and of the role your treatment has played in the client's recovery.

Next, you start all over again. List the client's current symptoms. Include everything the client can no longer do, or can no longer do without aggravating the symptoms. State also your current objective findings. Discuss the residual symptoms and test results in light of what is commonly expected of soft tissue injuries or disease. Include any adaptations that must occur in treatment and in the activities of daily life during periods when the symptoms are exacerbated.

Often your prognosis is requested. If it is, include your opinion regarding the probable cause of this client's symptomology. State your opinion regarding the expected soft tissue recovery time and completeness. Give an estimate regarding future treatment needed to maintain the current level of health. Close by offering yourself and your time for further questions. Remember not to give your opinion unless it is specifically requested. Any form of diagnosis is outside the scope of practice for a Licensed Massage Practitioner.

If the narrative is written to inform another caregiver, you will summarize the information from a single status report rather than the entire file. The SOAP format is still used. Summarize the subjective and objective information of the previous report and compare it to the current subjective and objective data. Assessment is the main focus in these narratives. Briefly present your proposed plan for continued treatments and a request for another prescription reflecting your plan, if necessary.

A sample narrative is as follows:

Ms. Ideal Client was first seen in my office on 4-17-92. She was referred by Dr. L.Y. Bones, D.C., with a diagnosis of an acceleration cervical injury with concommittant TMJ and low back strain as a result of an MVA on 4-15-92. The initial prescription included massage therapy and hydrotherapy treatments twice a week.

Ms. Client describes the onset of the accident as follows: It was a rainy day in Seattle. She was driving a compact car and was rear-ended by a station wagon while stopped at a red light. She was wearing a shoulder harness and lap belt, and notes that her headrest leans backward and cannot be elevated. Ms. Client's car was in neutral with no brake on, which allowed the wagon to push her into the intersection at considerable speed.

INITIAL SYMPTOMS:

Client initially presented herself with the following complaints:

1. *Severe headaches, constant since DOI.*

2. *Moderate neck pain and stiffness, constant, increasing in severity with reading, driving, exercise, and housework.*

3. *Moderate jaw pain intermittent since DOI, occurs with eating, clenching and grinding. Wakes up with jaw pain.*

4. *Restless sleep due to pain since DOI.*

5. *Inability to do normal duties including lifting, cleaning, working, gardening, running or aerobics since DOI.*

Client began complaining of the following symptoms two to three weeks post injury:

1. *Low back pain mild constant increasing in severity with prolonged sitting or standing, lifting or increase in activity.*

2. *Severe shooting pain down the left leg, intermittent with standing up from a seated position.*

INITIAL FINDINGS:

Upon examination the following objective findings were noted:

1. *Moderate hypertonicities: Bilateral scalenes, Splenius group, Pectoralis major and minor.*

2. *Moderate to severe spasms: Bilateral Sternocleidomastoid, Trapezius, Rhomboids, Erector spinae, Quadratus Lumborum, Masseter.*

3. *ROM moderate decrease in passive ROM with moderate pain in flexion, lateral flexion and rotation bilaterally. Too painful to test extension.*

4. *Posture - bilateral shoulder elevation with internal rotation, Left hip elevation with internal rotation.*

5. *Breathing - shallow with pain on deep inhalation.*

6. *Acute inflammation - redness, heat and swelling mid paracervical region and lumbo-sacral region.*

7. *Moderate pain with digital pressure in the neck shoulders, and low back regions.*

TREATMENT:

Initial treatment consisted of Manual Lymphatic Drainage to the neck and back to decrease inflammation. Ice was suggested as homework to continue the process of reducing inflammation and pain. Swedish massage and Polarity was applied to the whole body to relax the muscle spasms and decrease the energy blockage. A total body approach was adopted to encourage the body to reach a state of balance to support the body in healing itself. This approach also was used to decrease the possibility of compensational holding patterns setting up in the supporting structures.

Once Ms. Client was out of the acute stage of inflammation various treatment techniques were utilized on the injured structures. Cross fiber friction was applied to the scar tissue forming. This technique is used to break up the formation of collagen fibers to decrease the possibility of adhesions and increase the function of the injured soft tissue. Passive stretching followed all applications of cross fiber friction to realign the scar tissue along the lines of stress.

Trigger point therapy was applied to the tender points. Applying direct pressure to tender points decreases the referred pain in other locations. This also aids in reducing spasms.

Muscle Energy Technique was used on shortened muscles to increase range of motion and function. This technique uses resistive Swedish gymnastics to reset the proprioceptors of the muscles simply to remind them how long they are. This also aids in decreasing the hypertonic muscles and in decreasing adhesions. Active Swedish gymnastics were suggested as homework to continue lengthening the tight muscles and mobilizing the joints.

Cranio-sacral therapy and breathing exercises were applied to strengthen the body's natural rhythms, break up adhesions and encourage nutritional flow throughout the entire body.

Massage sessions began at two times weekly, tapered down to weekly after three months, and currently sessions are twice monthly. When her periodic exacerbations occur, the frequency of treatment increases to weekly sessions. Ms. Client has been showing steady improvement, but continues to experience persistent dysfunction in her neck and back with any excess of activity. This excess of activity today is still not consistent with what was considered normal activity for her before the motor vehicle accident.

CURRENT STATUS:

Currently Ms. Client's subjective findings include the following:

1. Headaches, moderate, lasting for 3-4 hours occurring after long periods of sitting, reading, driving, or with heavy stress.

2. Neck and shoulder pain and stiffness, mild, constant, increasing as day progresses.

3. Low back pain, mild, intermittent, occurs with sitting, standing, lifting.

4. Able to participate fully in life but with many restrictions, activities limited to short time spans, any strenuous activity causes pain immediately and she "pays for it" the next day with stiffness and pain.

5. TMJ pain infrequent, mild, only occurring with clenching and grinding at night after very stressful days or over exertion.

Client's current objective findings include the following:

1. *Hypertonicities: mild, bilateral scalenes, sternocleidomastoid, trapezius, pectoralis minor, erector spinae, and masseter. Left quadratus lumborum, external rotators, and psoas.*

2. *ROM: mild hypermobile bilateral cervical rotation and flexion with mild pain, mild hypomobile bilateral extention and lateral flexion with mild pain.*

3. *Adhesions and trigger points in neck and low back regions.*

Ms. Client's sleeping patterns have returned to normal, the spasms are infrequent, the shooting pain down the left leg has subsided, only to recur with periodic exacerbations. She has returned to normal duty at work and has begun participating in her normal household duties. She has not returned to her normal exercise program of running and weight-lifting. Her free time is considerably shorter as it takes her longer to perform her normal activities and she requires a lengthy daily stretching and strengthening program just to maintain her current ability to function.

Client's symptoms are, in my opinion, a direct result of the motor vehicle accident on 4-15-92. Due to the nature of soft tissue injuries, Ms. Client may expect to continue to experience periodic exacerbations of her symptoms for an undetermined length of time. Once muscle tissue is damaged it is never the same again. Bone tissue, for example, heals with calcium, a product of bone, creating a bond as strong as if not stronger than it was before. Muscles heal with a foreign substance, leaving the tissue less elastic, less flexible, weaker and prone to re-injury. Where the damage occurred, Ms. Client's soft tissue will never be as good as it was before.

Ms. Client will require daily stretching and strengthening, and monthly massage therapy, increasing to weekly with any exacerbations, to maintain her current condition, as per the doctor's recommendation. If you have any questions, or need to consult me further, please call.

Yours In Health,

The Best Hands In The West, LMP

NOTE:

Narrative reports, unlike other kinds of reports or charts, may be charged for if they are requested by an insurance company or an attorney. Send the bill to the party requesting the narrative **before** sending the report, to establish agreement for the requested document and for the charges. Often insurance companies will change their minds upon receipt of the bill and will then just request a copy of your client file in order to review your SOAP charts. Attorneys may pay you up front for your narrative reports. If this is the case, make sure you send your report immediately following receipt of payment.

Attorneys commonly request narrative reports to help substantiate a client's personal injury claim against an insurance company. Your documented information may be extremely valuable to the case even without primary care giver status. Attorneys are accustomed to paying for these services. The charge is ultimately absorbed by the client and usually comes out of the final settlement.

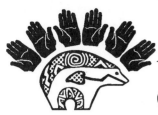

Chapter 8: *Professional Ethics*

Massage, in various forms, has been with us a long time. But the status of massage in our society has been changing dramatically over the past few decades. Massage is now increasingly seen as a valuable therapeutic tool for many types of injuries, and as a significant health-enhancing aid for everyone.

As public perceptions have changed, so have the training and status of massage practitioners. Therapeutic massage used to be the province of chiropractic assistants, physical therapy aides, and nurses—people with a background in medicine, but little or no training in massage therapy. Today's licensed massage practitioners (LMP's), however, learn not only the basics of health care, but are highly educated in anatomy, physiology, and kinesiology. Massage therapy **is** their specialty.

As a result, massage practitioners find themselves now in a slightly different relationship to physicians and to their clients than in the past. What follows are some guidelines regarding professional conduct for today's LMP.

THE DOCTOR AND YOU

As health care is currently structured, a physician or doctor (M.D., N.D., D.O., or D.C.) will be the **primary** caregiver. It is the doctor's responsibility to diagnose the client's problem and to orchestrate treatment.

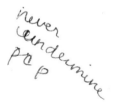

Since you are working at the doctor's direction but not under the doctor's supervision, good communication between you becomes essential. You must be sure that the primary caregiver has clear, complete information so that she or he can give the client the best possible treatment. Your SOAP charts will play an important part in this communication process.

Occasionally you may find yourself differing with a doctor about a client's condition or treatment. Do not express this disagreement to the client. Instead, state your views to the doctor—calmly, professionally, and tactfully, with all the supporting evidence you can provide. A doctor will generally give you a fair hearing if your documentation is good. If your input is not considered or if you find that you can't endorse the prescribed treatment, your best choice may be to withdraw from the case.

However you choose to handle the situation, remember that the primary caregiver is the final authority, and that it is unethical for the massage practitioner to undermine the relationship between the primary caregiver and the client.

THE CLIENT AND YOU

There are several things to remember about your relationship with your clients.

The first thing to remember, of course, is that your clients deserve your respect. Many clients may have had the experience of being treated impersonally or condescendingly by health providers. You must make it clear that you see the client as a person, not as a collection of symptoms, and as a participant in the healing process.

Second, keep in mind the probability that your client is suffering some degree of cognitive impairment. This will obviously be the case where concussion is involved, but even in cases where there is no head injury you may find a client's mental function to be reduced by chronic pain or by post-traumatic stress syndrome. Be patient if the client seems easily confused; make your questions and explanations as clear and simple as possible.

Third, remember that education is an important part of what you do. Some clients will already know a great deal about health matters, but many will need some basic information about the inter-relationship of body systems and about the relationship of body to mind. (Happily, since Bill Moyers produced his PBS series on mind and body, public awareness of and interest in the subject are much increased.) Some clients will need to be guided to a better body awareness as well.

Fourth, be aware that psychological issues may come up that are outside the scope of your practice. Learn to to treat your clients with care and concern, but also with an appropriate degree of professional detachment. It is important, for example, to know that your client has a sedentary job and is currently finding work stressful. It is not necessary or appropriate for you to hear all the details about the job or about the office politics involved. Validate the client's feelings, but steer the conversation gently toward more general and less personal information. Any specifics that you do learn, of course, should be treated as "privileged communications", and should not be charted nor discussed with other caregivers.

Occasionally the bodywork you are doing will trigger very strong emotions. Keep the focus on the physical sensations associated with the emotions. This will help strengthen the mind-body connection. Also, be sure the client is seeing a therapist who can help him or her to sort these feelings out.

Your SOAP charts can be as useful a tool for your client as they are for you and the doctor. Explain tests as you do them. Tell your clients what you are writing on their charts. Let them know that they're making progress, and get them involved in the healing process. Use the charting process to build a bridge between your client and yourself, not to erect a clinical wall separating the two of you.

Lastly, keep sight of a broader context than healing short-term injuries or conditions. Help your clients to develop a better understanding of and relationship to their bodies. Help them to form new habits that will give them a lifetime of better health.

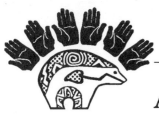

Appendix 1: *Abbreviations*

I. DESCRIPTIVE ADJECTIVES
1. L — mild, light
2. M — moderate
3. S — severe, significant
4. cons. — constant
5. freq. — frequent
6. inter. — intermittent
7. seld. — seldom

II. SYMPTOM
1. HA — headache
2. Ⓟ — pain
3. I, I-A, I-S, I-C — inflammation, acute, subacute, chronic
4. tp — tender point
5. Sp — spasm
6. ten. — tension

III. SYMBOLS
1. ∅ — none, no
2. c̄, w/ — with
3. s̄, w/o — without
4. ā, pre — before
5. p, post — after
6. ↑ — increase
7. ↓ — decrease
8. △ — change
9. 2° — due to, as a result of
10. ↻ — rotation
11. X — times
12. > — greater than
13. < — less than
14. → — through ie. 1 → 7, leads to, results in
15. +, - — positive, negative; plus, minus

IV. MASSAGE TERMS/TECHNIQUES
1. XFF — cross fiber friction *TFM transverse fiber friction massage*
2. DP — direct pressure
3. LD — lymphatic drainage *MLD manual lymphatic drainage*
4. Sw. Ⓜ — swedish massage
5. Ⓜ — massage
6. lin. F — linear friction *PFF parallel fiber friction*
7. MET — muscle energy technique *(PIR & RI)*
8. SCS — strain counter-strain
9. Pol. — polarity
10. PNF — proprioceptive neuromuscular facilitation
11. C/S — cranial-sacral therapy
12. NMT — neuromuscular therapy
13. MFR — myofascial release
14. STM — soft tissue manipulation
15. MLD — manual lymphatic drainage

V. DIRECTIONS

1.	Ⓛ	left
2.	Ⓡ	right
3.	BL	bilateral
4.	sup.	superior
5.	inf.	inferior
6.	ant.	anterior
7.	post.	posterior
8.	med.	medial
9.	lat.	lateral
10.	caud.	caudal
11.	ceph.	cephalic
12.	prox.	proximal
13.	dist.	distal
14.	int.	internal
15.	ext.	external
16.	prone	prone
17.	sup.	supine
18.	SL	side lying

Spell out (handwritten note pointing to 17–18)

VI. ACTIONS

1.	ROM	range of motion
2.	A, P, R-ROM	active, passive, resistive
3.	add.	adduction
4.	abd.	abduction
5.	rot.	rotation
6.	flex.	flexion
7.	ext.	extension
8.	sup.	supination
9.	pron.	pronation
10.	~~SB~~ *Lat. Flex*	side bending *Lateral Flexion*
11.	inv.	inversion
12.	evr.	eversion
13.	uln./rad. dev.	ulnar/radial deviation
14.	protr.	protraction
15.	retr.	retraction
16.	WNL	within normal limits *(find out what this means)*

VII. LOCATIONS- GENERAL EXAMPLES- FOLLOW SUIT WITH ANY OTHERS BY SHORTENING THE WORD

1.	C-1 → 7	cervical vertebrae 1 thru 7
2.	T-1 → 12	thoracic vertebrae 1 thru 12
3.	L-1 → 5	lumbar vertebrae 1 thru 5
4.	paravert,paracerv...	around/attaching to the vertebrae
5.	TVP, *TP*	transverse process
6.	SP	spinous process
7.	ITB	illio-tibial band
8.	SI	sacro-illiac
9.	LB	low back

Spell out (handwritten note pointing to 9)

	10. QL	quadratus lumborum
	11. SCM	sternocleidomastoid
	12. lats	latissimus dorsi
	13. traps	trapezius
	14. delt	deltoid
	15. pec	pectoralis
	16. mj+m	major and minor
	17. lev. scap.	levator scapulae
	18. gastroc.	gastrocnemius
VIII. MEDICAL RECORDS/MISC./ PRESCRIPTIONS	1. Tx	treatment
	2. Hx	history
	3. Rx	prescription
	4. Dx	diagnosis
	5. Px	prognosis
	6. NA	non-applicable
	7. c/o	complains of
	8. mm	muscle
	9. pt	patient
	10. DOI	date of injury
	11. MVA	motor vehicle accident
	12. meds	medication
	13. OTC	over the counter
	14. PRN	as necessary/ as needed
	15. qd	every day
	16. bid	twice a day
	17. tid	three times a day
	18. qid	four times a day
	19. qod	every other day
	20. ac	before meals
	21. pc	after meals
	22. qhs	at bedtime
	23. po	orally
	24. pr	rectally
	25. iv	intravenous
	26. sc	subcutaneous
	27. im	intramuscular
	28. IME	"independent" medical exam
	29. PA	postural analysis
	30. ER	emergency room
	Ax	assesment

IX. HEALTH CARE PROVIDERS	1.	LMP	licensed massage practitioner
	2.	PT	physical therapist
	3.	DC	doctor of chiropractic
	4.	DO	doctor of osteopathy
	5.	MD	medical doctor
	6.	RN	registered nurse
	7.	LPN	licensed practical nurse
	8.	ND	naturopathic doctor
	9.	MSW	masters in social work
	10.	CDC	chemical dependency counselor
	11.	OT	occupational therapist
	12.	RT	recreational therapist
	13.	HCA	health care assistant
	14.	ARNP	accredited registered nurse practitioner

X. MALADIES	1.	HA	headache
	2.	HT	hypertonicity
	3.	TP	trigger point
	4.	Adh.	adhesion
	5.	OA	osteoarthritis
	6.	RA	rheumatoid arthritis
	7.	str.	strain
	8.	spr.	sprain
	9.	Fx	fracture
	10.	PTS	post-traumatic stress syndrome
	11.	CFS	chronic fatigue syndrome
	12.	MS	multiple sclerosis
	13.	CP	cerebral palsy
	14.	AC sep.	acromio-clavicular separation
	15.	scol.	scoliosis
	16.	lord.	lordosis
	17.	kyph.	kyphosis
	18.	CTS	carpal tunnel syndrome
	19.	TOS	thoracic outlet syndrome
	20.	FM	fibromyalgia

Handwritten annotations: Spell out (linking items 5–9); hyper or hypo — (linking items 16 & 17)

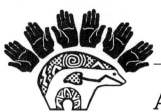

Appendix 2: *Case Study*

The following is a sample case study of a client diagnosed with an acceleration/deceleration cervical injury and concomitant TMJ and low back strain.

Included are all initial intake forms, an initial status report, four SOAP charts, and a status update. These charts are representative of the narrative report presented in chapter seven.

BLANK FORMS AVAILABLE FOR SALE

Please note that all forms contained in this case study, with the exception of the "Vernon-Minor/revised Oswestry" form, are **copyrighted by the author** and may not be reproduced in any form without written permission of the author.

If you are interested in purchasing any blank forms contained in this case study, please contact the author.

Diana L. Thompson, L.M.P.
Healing Arts Studio
916 N.E. 64th
Seattle, Washington 98115

INITIAL INJURY INFORMATION

Name: __Ms. Ideal Client__   Date of Onset: __4·15·92__

Description of Onset: __pt. rear-ended   MVA__
__pt. driving compact - hit by station wagon ~ 20 mph__
__pt. stopped at red light, car in neutral, no brake on__
__car forced into intersection upon impact - wet roads__
__pt. wearing seat belt / sh. harness, headrest below__
__center of gravity of head + tilts backward - no resting__
__contact__
__pt. facing forward upon impact__

Primary Symptoms:

Rate symptom intensity "mild", "moderate", "severe"

S HA
M neck Ⓟ + stiffness
M jaw Ⓟ
restless sleep

List all symptoms immediately post injury: __nausea, diziness, ringing in ears - 24 hrs.__
__achey feeling all over__

List all other associated symptoms prior to today: __none__

(AUTHOR'S NOTE: This is valuable information when the time between the

DOI and the first date of tx is extensive.)

What physical duties are required for your job? __Sitting at computer for hours__

What regular activities of daily living are affected by this injury? __housework, gardening, reading,__
__driving, running, lifting__

List all adjunctive therapies received for this injury: __chiropractic , ER - admitted and__
__released w/in 4 hrs. post exam + X-rays__

Insurance &/or attorney information: __Cars·R·us policy # 1234567 adjuster: Enid__
__attorney: Richard Adler   paralegal: Barbara__

To whom should treatment billing be sent? __Adler Giersch PS attn. Barbara__
__401 2nd Ave. S. Suite 600 Seattle, Wa 98104 206·682·0300__

PERSONAL HEALTH INFORMATION

PERSONAL DATA

Name: __Ms. Ideal Client__   Date: __4-17-92__   Referred by: __Dr. LY Bones__

Address: __1313 Mockingbird LN.__   Phone - Day: __555-9889__

City/State/Zip: __Crab Apple Cove, WA. 98126__   Phone - Eve: __555-8338__

Birthday: __5.31.60__   Occupation/Employer: __Stats Processor - Seattle Mariners__

Primary Health Care Provider: __Dr. LY Bones__   Phone: __555-1991__

Permission to consult with primary provider? Please initial if yes. ☒ Yes __IC__   ☐ No

Emergency contact: __Mary Lou Hostetter__   Phone: __555-3260__

MASSAGE HISTORY/TREATMENT INFORMATION

Have you ever received a professional massage? ☒ Yes ☐ No If yes, frequency __occasional__ Date of last massage __2.14.92__

What results do you want from your massage sessions? __pain relief, relaxation, more movement__

Prioritze the areas of your body that you would prefer to be massaged. __neck - be careful!__
__jaw + back__
__feet please!__

Please check the areas of your body that you give permission to receive massage:
☒ back ☒ legs ☒ buttocks ☒ arms ☒ abdomen ☒ chest ☒ neck ☒ head ☒ face ☒ other __feet__

Are you currently seeing a medical practitioner? Please explain if yes. ☒ Yes ☐ No __D.C. for MVA__

Are you currently seeing a psychotherapist or are you attending regular support group meetings? Please explain if yes. ☒ Yes ☐ No
__weekly CODA mtgs.__

List stress reduction and exercise activities. Include frequency. __running + weight lifting 3x/wk__
__rowing, cycling, skiing seasonally__

List current medications, including aspirin, ibuprofen, etc. __Advil 4x/dy 800 mg.__
__Synthroid 2 mg/dy__

PREVIOUS HISTORY (Include year and treatment received)

Surgeries: __C-section July 1990__
__arthroscopy (R) knee Sept. '87__
__pins in (L) hand Feb. '82__
Accidents: __prior MVA Feb. '82 broken hand pinned/surgery__
__(L) sh tear winter '83 no tx pain pills__
__multiple head injuries - rugby '80-'88 no tx pain pills__
__skiing accident (R) knee tear potential for surgery__

HEALTH HISTORY

MUSCULO-SKELETAL

_____ bone or joint disease _____

_____ tendonitis _____

_____ bursitis _____

✓ broken/fractured bones ___ Ⓛ hand _____

_____ arthritis _____

✓ sprains/strains __ ankles, sh Ⓛ, knee Ⓡ __

_____ low back, hip, leg pain _____

✓ neck, shoulder, arm pain __ current ____

✓ headaches/head injuries __ current / multiple __

✓ spasms/cramps __ current - neck + back __

✓ jaw pain/TMJ __ current ____

_____ lupus _____

_____ other _____

CIRCULATORY

_____ heart condition _____

✓ varicose veins __ Ⓛ leg - back·side __

_____ blood clots _____

_____ high blood pressure _____

_____ low blood pressure _____

_____ lymphedema _____

_____ breathing difficulty _____

_____ sinus problems _____

✓ allergies __ cats , lima beans __

_____ other _____

INFECTIOUS DISEASE

_____ disease name(s): _____

_____

_____

SKIN

_____ allergies _____

_____ rashes _____

_____ athletes foot _____

_____ warts _____

_____ other _____

DIGESTIVE

✓ constipation __ w/ mensus + pizza __

_____ gas/bloating _____

_____ diverticulitis _____

_____ irritable bowel syndrome _____

_____ other _____

NERVOUS SYSTEM

_____ herpes/shingles _____

_____ numbness/tingling _____

_____ chronic pain _____

_____ fatigue _____

✓ sleep disorders __ current __

_____ other _____

REPRODUCTIVE

_____ pregnant? Stage _____

✓ PMS __ moody , HA, cramps __

_____ other _____

OTHER

_____ cancer/tumors _____

_____ diabetes _____

_____ eating disorders _____

_____ depression _____

_____ drug/alcohol addiction _____

✓ nicotine/caffeine addiction __ espresso __

It is my choice to receive massage therapy. I realize that the treatment is being given for the well-being of my body and mind. This includes stress reduction, relief from muscular tension, spasm or pain, or for increasing circulation or energy flow. I agree to communicate with my practitioner any time I feel like my well being is being compromised.

I understand that massage practitioners do not diagnose illness, disease, or any physical or mental disorder; nor do they prescribe medical treatment, pharmaceuticals, or perform spinal thrust manipulations. I acknowledge that massage is not a substitute for medical examination or diagnosis, and that it is recommended that I see a primary health care provider for that service.

I have stated all medical conditions that I am aware of and will update the massage practitioner of any changes in my health status.

SIGNATURE: _Ideal Client_   DATE: _4·17·92_

Name: **Ms. Ideal Client**   Date: **4-17-92**

This questionnaire has been designed to give the health care provider information as to how your neck pain has affected your ability to manage everyday life. Please answer every section and mark in each section only the **ONE** box which applies to you. We realize you may consider that two of the statements in any one section relate to you, but please just mark the box which most closely describes your problem today.

SECTION 1- PAIN INTENSITY
- ☐ I have no pain at the moment.
- ☐ The pain is very mild at the moment.
- ☐ The pain is moderate at the moment.
- ☒ The pain is fairly severe at the moment.
- ☐ The pain is very severe at the moment.
- ☐ The pain is the worst imaginable at the moment.

SECTION 2- PERSONAL CARE (washing, dressing etc.)
- ☐ I can look after myself normally without causing pain.
- ☐ I can look after myself normally but it causes extra pain.
- ☒ It is painful to look after myself and I am slow and careful.
- ☐ I need some help but manage most of my personal care.
- ☐ I need help every day in most aspects of self care.
- ☐ I do not get dressed, I wash with difficulty and I stay in bed.

SECTION 3- LIFTING
- ☐ I can lift heavy weights without extra pain.
- ☐ I can lift heavy weights but it gives extra pain.
- ☐ Pain prevents me from lifting heavy weights off the floor, but I can manage if they are conveniently positioned, for example on a table.
- ☒ Pain prevents me from lifting heavy weights, but I can manage light to medium weights if they are conveniently positioned.
- ☐ I can lift very light weights.
- ☐ I cannot lift or carry anything at all.

SECTION 4- READING
- ☐ I can read as much as I want to with no pain in my neck.
- ☐ I can read as much as I want to with slight pain in my neck.
- ☐ I can read as much as I want to with moderate pain in my neck.
- ☐ I can't read as much as I want because of moderate pain in my neck.
- ☒ I can hardly read at all because of severe pain in my neck.
- ☐ I cannot read at all.

SECTION 5- HEADACHES
- ☐ I have no headaches at all.
- ☐ I have slight headaches which come infrequently.
- ☐ I have moderate headaches which come infrequently.
- ☐ I have moderate headaches which come frequently.
- ☒ I have severe headaches which come frequently.
- ☐ I have headaches almost all of the time.

SECTION 6- CONCENTRATION
- ☐ I can concentrate fully when I want to with no difficulty.
- ☐ I can concentrate fully when I want to with slight difficulty.
- ☐ I have a fair degree of difficulty in concentrating when I want to.
- ☒ I have a great deal of difficulty in concentrating when I want to.
- ☐ I cannot concentrate at all.

SECTION 7- WORK
- ☐ I can do as much work as I want to.
- ☐ I can do my usual work but no more.
- ☐ I can do most of my usual work but no more.
- ☒ I cannot do my usual work.
- ☐ I can hardly do any work at all.
- ☐ I can't do any work at all.

SECTION 8- DRIVING
- ☐ I can drive my car without any neck pain.
- ☐ I can drive my car as long as I want with slight pain in my neck.
- ☐ I can drive my car as long as I want with moderate pain in my neck.
- ☐ I can't drive my car as long as I want because of moderate pain in my neck.
- ☒ I can hardly drive at all because of severe pain in my neck.
- ☐ I can't drive my car at all.

SECTION 9- SLEEPING
- ☐ I have no trouble sleeping.
- ☐ My sleep is slightly disturbed (less than one hour sleepless).
- ☐ My sleep is mildly disturbed (1-2 hrs. sleepless).
- ☒ My sleep is moderately disturbed (2-3 hrs. sleepless).
- ☐ My sleep is greatly disturbed (3-5 hrs. sleepless).
- ☐ My sleep is completely disturbed (5-7 hrs. sleepless).

SECTION 10- RECREATION.
- ☐ I am able to engage in all my recreation activities with no neck pain at all.
- ☐ I am able to engage in all my recreation activities, with some pain in my neck.
- ☐ I am able to engage in most, but not all of my usual recreation activities because of pain in my neck.
- ☐ I am able to engage in a few of my usual recreation activities because of pain in my neck.
- ☒ I hardly do any recreation activities because of pain in my neck.
- ☐ I can't do recreation activities at all.

PERSONAL STATUS REPORT

Name: __Ms. Ideal Client__   Date: __4·17·92__

Identify **CURRENT** symptomatic areas in your body by drawing the symbols on the figures below.

KEY: ◯   Circle areas of **PAIN**

X   "X" over areas of **JOINT AND MUSCLE STIFFNESS**

≶   Draw a squiggly lines along the areas of **NUMBNESS OR TINGLING**

╫   Mark **SCARS, BRUISES** or **OPEN WOUNDS**

Additional comments: __Various veins - Ⓛ leg - Varicose__

_____

_____

_____

_____

_____

CURRENT MEDS Advil qid , synthroid

S

CLIENT GOALS / UPDATE

↓ Ⓟ ↓ spasms ↑ rest

LOCATION / SYMPTOMS / INTENSITY / FREQUENCY / DURATION / ONSET

HA Ⓟ S cons. post DOI - MVA

neck Ⓟ, M "   "   "   "
  stiffness

jaw Ⓟ M interm. "   "   "

Ⓟ preventing restful sleep

AGGRAVATING / RELIEVING CIRCUMSTANCES REGARDING ACTIVITIES OF DAILY LIVING

A: driving, sitting, standing, reading, lifting,
   exercise, housework, childcare

R: ice, advil, chiro. adj.

O

HYPERTONICITIES-INTENSITY, VISUAL / PALPABLE OBSERVATIONS, ADDITIONAL TESTS

I - red, heat, swell. - paracerv.

spasms BL - M - scms, traps, rhomb., QL,
            erec. sp., masseter

HT BL - M - scalenes, splen. grp., Pecs mj+m

Breathing - shallow - Ⓟ w/ deep inhal.

TREATMENT GOALS

↓ Ⓟ ↓ I ↓ Sp. ↓ HT ↑ energy ↑ relax.

MASSAGE

Sw Ⓜ + Pol. - arms, legs
   Supine: pillows + ice - cerv.
        MLD neck + chest
        pressure pts. face, jaw, head
        reflex - feet
        nerve strokes

A

CHANGES DUE TO MASSAGE

↓ I - M Δ

↓ HT - L Δ overall ↑ Rom lat flex L Δ

↓ Sp - L Δ neck ⌀ LB M Δ jaw

↓ Ⓟ M → L+ neck ⌀ LB M → L - jaw

↓ HA S → M

↑ bal / relax overall

P

SUGGESTED TREATMENT PLAN

2x wk / 4 wk - re·eval 5.13 per 'script.

P·Rom cerv. avail. next tx.

HOMEWORK

ice packs 2-3 x/dy neck or prn

↑ short rest periods

_____BHW_____ , LMP

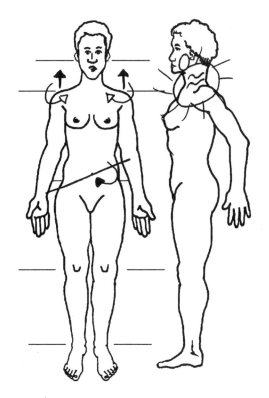

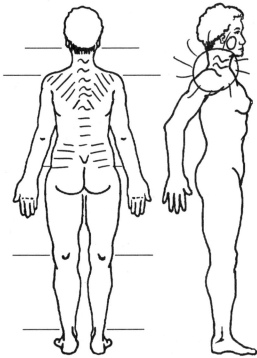

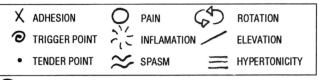

X ADHESION	O PAIN	↻ ROTATION	
℗ TRIGGER POINT	☼ INFLAMATION	/ ELEVATION	
• TENDER POINT	≈ SPASM	= HYPERTONICITY	

© DIANA L. THOMPSON, 1993 NO. 01

NAME Ms. Ideal Client **DATE** 4·17·92

RANGE OF MOTION		ACTIVE		
*No Right or Left evaluation	ROM		PAIN	
SPINAL	R	L	R	L
TRUNK SIDEBENDING				
TRUNK ROTATION				
EXTENSION *				
FLEXION *				

K E Y	WNL	Within Normal Limits	↑	Hypermobility
	L	Mild	↓	Hypomobility
	M	Moderate	P	Pain
	S	Severe	Ⓟ	No Pain

RANGE OF MOTION	ACTIVE				PASSIVE				RESISTED			
	ROM		PAIN		ROM		PAIN		STRENGTH		PAIN	
HIP	R	L	R	L	R	L	R	L	R	L	R	L
FLEXION												
EXTENSION												
ABDUCTION												
ADDUCTION												
INTERNAL ROTATION												
EXTERNAL ROTATION												
NECK	R	L	R	L	R	L	R	L	R	L	R	L
FLEXION *	↓M		M		↓M		M		↓M		M	
EXTENSION *	too much mm guarding				too Ⓟful to test				↓M		M	
LATERAL FLEXION	↓M	↓M	M	M	↓M	↓M	M	M	WNL	WNL	Ⓟ	Ⓟ
ROTATION	↓L	↓L	L	L	↓M	↓M	M	M	WNL	WNL	Ⓟ	Ⓟ
SHOULDER	R	L	R	L	R	L	R	L	R	L	R	L
FLEXION												
EXTENSION												
ABDUCTION												
ADDUCTION												
HORIZONTAL ADDUCTION												
HORIZONTAL ABDUCTION												
INTERNAL ROTATION												
EXTERNAL ROTATION												
PAINFUL ARC												
KNEE	R	L	R	L	R	L	R	L	R	L	R	L
FLEXION												
EXTENSION												
INTERNAL ROTATION												
EXTERNAL ROTATION												
VALGUS												
VARUS												
ANTERIOR DRAWER												
POSTERIOR DRAWER												
ANKLE	R	L	R	L	R	L	R	L	R	L	R	L
DORSIFLEXION												
PLANTARFLEXION												
INVERSION												
EVERSION												
SUPINATION												
PRONATION												
ADDUCTION												
ABDUCTION												
OTHER	R	L	R	L	R	L	R	L	R	L	R	L

NAME **Ms. Ideal Client**   DATE **5-5-92**

DOI **4.15.92**   CURRENT MEDS **Advil qid   synthroid**

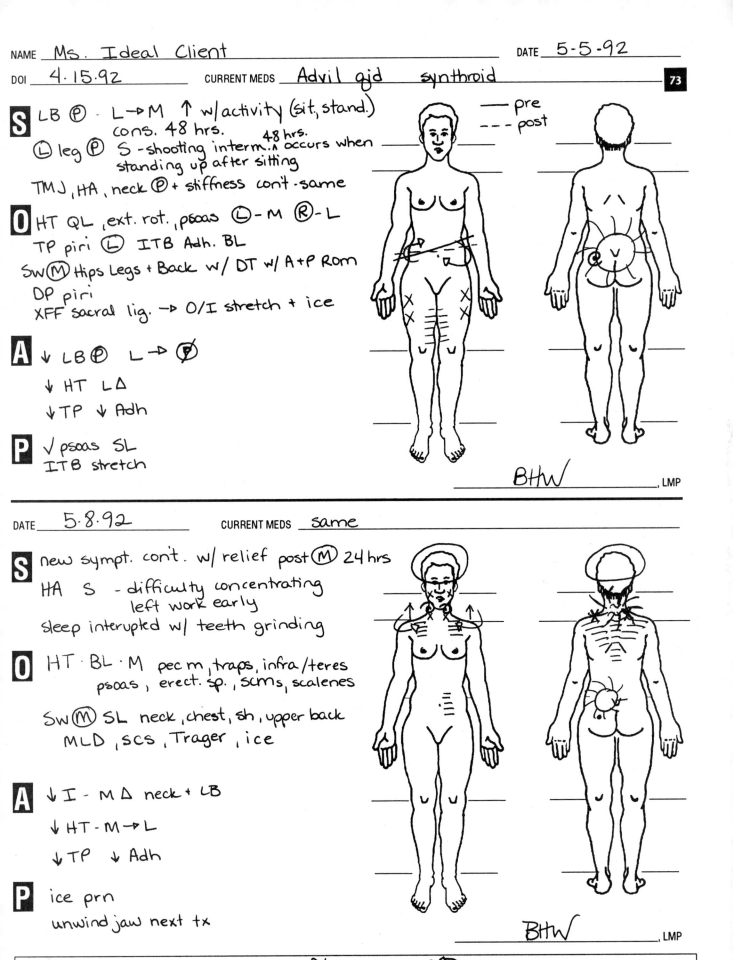

S LB Ⓟ · L→M ↑ w/activity (sit, stand.)
　　cons. 48 hrs.
　Ⓛ leg Ⓟ S -shooting interm. 48 hrs. occurs when
　　standing up after sitting
　TMJ, HA, neck Ⓟ + stiffness cont · same

O HT QL, ext. rot., psoas Ⓛ-M Ⓡ-L
　TP piri Ⓛ ITB Adh. BL
　Sw Ⓜ hips Legs + Back w/ DT w/ A+P Rom
　DP piri
　XFF sacral lig. → O/I stretch + ice

A ↓ LB Ⓟ L→ Ⓟ
　↓ HT L△
　↓ TP ↓ Adh

P √ psoas SL
　ITB stretch

_____ , LMP **BHW**

DATE **5.8.92**   CURRENT MEDS **same**

S new sympt. cont. w/ relief post Ⓜ 24 hrs
　HA S - difficulty concentrating
　　　left work early
　sleep interupted w/ teeth grinding

O HT · BL · M pec m, traps, infra/teres
　　psoas, erect. sp., scms, scalenes
　Sw Ⓜ SL neck, chest, sh, upper back
　　MLD, scs, Trager, ice

A ↓ I - M △ neck + LB
　↓ HT - M→L
　↓ TP ↓ Adh

P ice prn
　unwind jaw next tx

_____ , LMP **BHW**

X	ADHESION	•	TENDER POINT	INFLAMATION	ᏻꝰ	ROTATION	≡	HYPERTONICITY
℗	TRIGGER POINT	O	PAIN	≈ SPASM	/	ELEVATION		© DIANA L. THOMPSON, 1993 NO. 02

NAME **Ms. Ideal Client**　　　　　　　DATE **7·5·92**

DOI **4·15·92**　　CURRENT MEDS **Advil prn**

S Drove 6 hrs. yest. = ↑ Symp
HA Ⓟ M cons. since yest.
Neck, Back, Sh Ⓟ + stiff M
cons. since yest., shooting Ⓟ Ⓛ leg

O mm guarding entire back, neck, sh, chest
I - neck + back S
↓ Rom A+P cerv. lat flex + rot.
　　　　LB spine SB + rot.
VF - 3cold 1 hot - 20 min.
FB - SW Ⓜ w/ Pol.
Still Pts feet - chaotic rhythm

A ↓ mm guarding
↑ bal. rhythm + energy MΔ
↓ I neck + LB
posture ΔL

P lumbar support for car
MLD next tx

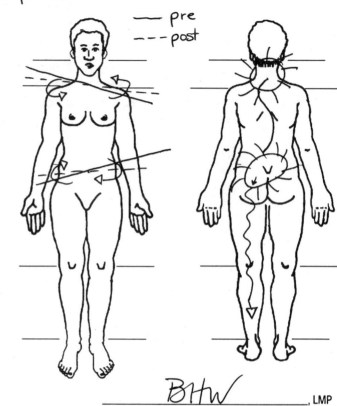

　　　　— pre
　　　- - - post

BHW　　　　　　, LMP

DATE **7·12·92**　　CURRENT MEDS **same**

S general improv. sleep
↓ symp 4 days post tx
all symp. L interm.
　(HA, neck, LB jaw Ⓟ + stiff.)

O neck congestion - multiple tender pts.
HT BL M scalenes, scms, lev. scap.
　　trap., pecs
Supine:
　LD - upper body
　C/S - unwinding - mandible
　XFF - scalenes / stretch, DP lev scap
　Legs - jost., reflex

A ↑ Rom TMJ MΔ
↓ congest. MΔ
↓ Adh
↓ + pts.

P self Ⓜ TMJ
status next tx

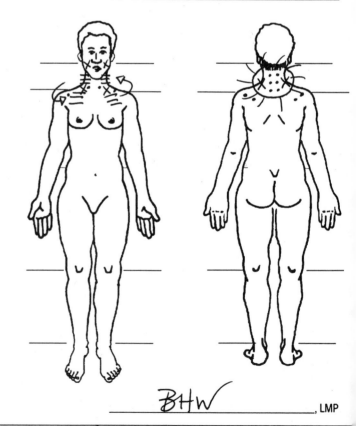

BHW　　　　　　, LMP

X	ADHESION	•	TENDER POINT	⚡	INFLAMATION	⟳	ROTATION	≡	HYPERTONICITY
⟲	TRIGGER POINT	O	PAIN	≈	SPASM	/	ELEVATION		© DIANA L. THOMPSON, 1993 NO. 02

Name: __Ms. Ideal Client__   Date: __1.22.93__

This questionnaire has been designed to give the health care provider information as to how your neck pain has affected your ability to manage everyday life. Please answer every section and mark in each section only the **ONE** box which applies to you. We realize you may consider that two of the statements in any one section relate to you, but please just mark the box which most closely describes your problem today.

SECTION 1- PAIN INTENSITY
- ☐ I have no pain at the moment.
- ☒ The pain is very mild at the moment.
- ☐ The pain is moderate at the moment.
- ☐ The pain is fairly severe at the moment.
- ☐ The pain is very severe at the moment.
- ☐ The pain is the worst imaginable at the moment.

SECTION 2- PERSONAL CARE (washing, dressing etc.)
- ☒ I can look after myself normally without causing pain.
- ☐ I can look after myself normally but it causes extra pain.
- ☐ It is painful to look after myself and I am slow and careful.
- ☐ I need some help but manage most of my personal care.
- ☐ I need help every day in most aspects of self care.
- ☐ I do not get dressed, I wash with difficulty and I stay in bed.

SECTION 3- LIFTING
- ☐ I can lift heavy weights without extra pain.
- ☒ I can lift heavy weights but it gives extra pain.
- ☐ Pain prevents me from lifting heavy weights off the floor, but I can manage if they are conveniently positioned, for example on a table.
- ☐ Pain prevents me from lifting heavy weights, but I can manage light to medium weights if they are conveniently positioned.
- ☐ I can lift very light weights.
- ☐ I cannot lift or carry anything at all.

SECTION 4- READING
- ☐ I can read as much as I want to with no pain in my neck.
- ☐ I can read as much as I want to with slight pain in my neck.
- ☐ I can read as much as I want to with moderate pain in my neck.
- ☒ I can't read as much as I want because of moderate pain in my neck.
- ☐ I can hardly read at all because of severe pain in my neck.
- ☐ I cannot read at all.

SECTION 5- HEADACHES
- ☐ I have no headaches at all.
- ☐ I have slight headaches which come infrequently.
- ☒ I have moderate headaches which come infrequently.
- ☐ I have moderate headaches which come frequently.
- ☐ I have severe headaches which come frequently.
- ☐ I have headaches almost all of the time.

SECTION 6- CONCENTRATION
- ☒ I can concentrate fully when I want to with no difficulty.
- ☐ I can concentrate fully when I want to with slight difficulty.
- ☐ I have a fair degree of difficulty in concentrating when I want to.
- ☐ I have a great deal of difficulty in concentrating when I want to.
- ☐ I cannot concentrate at all.

SECTION 7- WORK
- ☐ I can do as much work as I want to.
- ☒ I can do my usual work but no more.
- ☐ I can do most of my usual work but no more.
- ☐ I cannot do my usual work.
- ☐ I can hardly do any work at all.
- ☐ I can't do any work at all.

SECTION 8- DRIVING
- ☐ I can drive my car without any neck pain.
- ☐ I can drive my car as long as I want with slight pain in my neck.
- ☐ I can drive my car as long as I want with moderate pain in my neck.
- ☒ I can't drive my car as long as I want because of moderate pain in my neck.
- ☐ I can hardly drive at all because of severe pain in my neck.
- ☐ I can't drive my car at all.

SECTION 9- SLEEPING
- ☒ I have no trouble sleeping.
- ☐ My sleep is slightly disturbed (less than one hour sleepless).
- ☐ My sleep is mildly disturbed (1-2 hrs. sleepless).
- ☐ My sleep is moderately disturbed (2-3 hrs. sleepless).
- ☐ My sleep is greatly disturbed (3-5 hrs. sleepless).
- ☐ My sleep is completely disturbed (5-7 hrs. sleepless).

SECTION 10- RECREATION.
- ☐ I am able to engage in all my recreation activities with no neck pain at all.
- ☐ I am able to engage in all my recreation activities, with some pain in my neck.
- ☒ I am able to engage in most, but not all of my usual recreation activities because of pain in my neck.
- ☐ I am able to engage in a few of my usual recreation activities because of pain in my neck.
- ☐ I hardly do any recreation activities because of pain in my neck.
- ☐ I can't do recreation activities at all.

LOW BACK PAIN AND DISABILITY QUESTIONNAIRE (revised Oswestry)

Name: _Ms. Ideal Client_   Date: _1·22·93_

This questionnaire has been designed to give the health care provider information as to how your back pain has affected your ability to manage everyday life. Please answer every section and mark in each section only the **ONE** box which applies to you. We realize you may consider that two of the statements in any one section relate to you, but please just mark the box which most closely describes your problem today.

SECTION 1- PAIN INTENSITY
- ☐ The pain comes and goes and is very mild.
- ☐ The pain is mild and does not vary much.
- ☒ The pain comes and goes and is moderate.
- ☐ The pain is moderate and does not vary much.
- ☐ The pain comes and goes and is very severe.
- ☐ The pain is severe and does not vary much.

SECTION 2- PERSONAL CARE
- ☒ I would not have to change my way of washing or dressing in order to avoid pain.
- ☐ I do not normally change my way of washing and dressing even though it causes some pain.
- ☐ Washing and dressing increase the pain but I manage not to change my way of doing it.
- ☐ Washing and dressing increase the pain and I find it necessary to change my way of doing it.
- ☐ Because of the pain I am unable to do some washing and dressing.
- ☐ Because of the pain I am unable to do any washing and dressing without help.

SECTION 3- LIFTING
- ☐ I can lift heavy weights without extra pain.
- ☒ I can lift heavy weights but it causes extra pain.
- ☐ Pain prevents me from lifting heavy weights off the floor.
- ☐ Pain prevents me from lifting heavy weights off the floor, but I manage if they are conveniently positioned (e.g. on a table).
- ☐ Pain prevents me from lifting heavy weights but I can manage light to medium weights if they are conveniently positioned.
- ☐ I can only lift very light weights at the most.

SECTION 4- WALKING
- ☐ I have no pain on walking.
- ☒ I have some pain on walking but it does not increase with distance.
- ☐ I cannot walk more than one mile without increasing pain.
- ☐ I cannot walk more than 1/2 mile without increasing pain.
- ☐ I cannot walk more than 1/4 mile without increasing pain.
- ☐ I cannot walk at all without increasing pain.

SECTION 5- SITTING
- ☐ I can sit in any chair as long as I like.
- ☒ I can only sit in my favorite chair as long as I like.
- ☐ Pain prevents me from sitting more than one hour.
- ☐ Pain prevents me from sitting more than 1/2 hour.
- ☐ Pain prevents me from sitting more than 10 minutes.
- ☐ I avoid sitting because it increases my pain straight away.

SECTION 6- STANDING
- ☐ I can stand as long as I want without pain.
- ☐ I have some pain on standing but it does not increase with time.
- ☒ I cannot stand for longer than one hour without increasing pain.
- ☐ I cannot stand for longer than 1/2 hour without increasing pain.
- ☐ I cannot stand for longer than 10 minutes without increasing pain.
- ☐ I avoid standing because it increases the pain straight away.

SECTION 7- SLEEPING
- ☒ I get no pain in bed.
- ☐ I get pain in bed but it does not prevent me from sleeping well.
- ☐ Because of pain my normal night's sleep is reduced by less than 1/4.
- ☐ because of pain my normal night's sleep is reduced by less than 1/2.
- ☐ Because of pain my normal night's sleep is reduced by less than 3/4.
- ☐ Pain prevents me from sleeping at all.

SECTION 8- SOCIAL LIFE
- ☐ My social life is normal and gives me no pain.
- ☐ My social life is normal but increases the degree of pain.
- ☒ Pain has no significant effect on my social life apart from limiting my more energetic interests, e.g. dancing, etc.
- ☐ Pain has restricted my social life and I do not go out very often.
- ☐ Pain has restricted my social to my home.
- ☐ I have hardly any social life because of the pain.

SECTION 9- TRAVELLING
- ☐ I get no pain whilst traveling.
- ☒ I get some pain whilst travelling but none of my usual forms of travel make it any worse.
- ☐ I get extra pain whilst travelling but it does not compel me to seek alternate forms of travel.
- ☐ I get extra pain whilst travelling which compels me to seek alternative forms of travel.
- ☐ Pain restricts all forms of travel.
- ☐ Pain prevents all forms of travel except that done lying down.

SECTION 10- CHANGING DEGREE OF PAIN
- ☐ My pain is rapidly getting better.
- ☒ My pain fluctuates but overall is definitely getting better.
- ☐ My pain seems to be getting better but improvement is slow at present.
- ☐ My pain is neither getting better or worse.
- ☐ My pain is gradually worsening.
- ☐ My pain is rapidly worsening.

PERSONAL STATUS REPORT

Name: __Ms. Ideal Client__   Date: __1·22·93__

Identify **CURRENT** symptomatic areas in your body by drawing the symbols on the figures below.

KEY:

◯   Circle areas of **PAIN**

✕   "X" over areas of **JOINT AND MUSCLE STIFFNESS**

〰   Draw a squiggly lines along the areas of **NUMBNESS OR TINGLING**

╫   Mark **SCARS, BRUISES** or **OPEN WOUNDS**

Additional comments: __pain and stiffness only present w/ activity__

NAME Ms. Ideal Client

DATE 1·22·93   **DOI** 4·15·92

CURRENT MEDS Ø , Synthroid

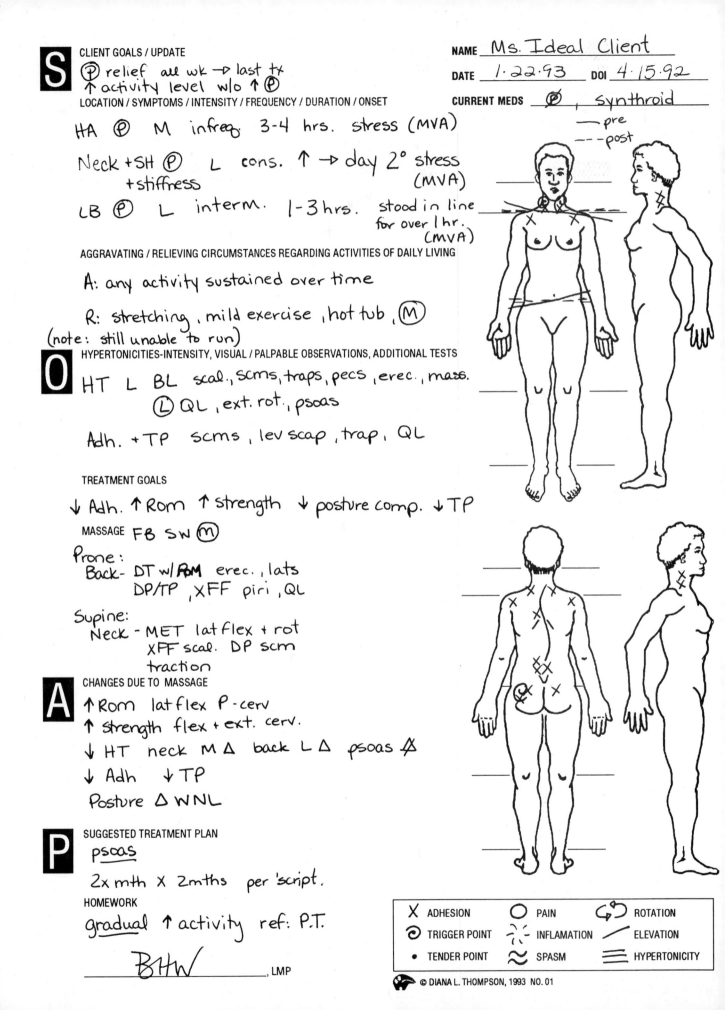

— pre
--- post

S — CLIENT GOALS / UPDATE

Ⓟ relief all wk → last tx
↑ activity level w/o ↑ Ⓟ

LOCATION / SYMPTOMS / INTENSITY / FREQUENCY / DURATION / ONSET

HA Ⓟ M infreq 3-4 hrs. stress (MVA)

Neck + SH Ⓟ L cons. ↑ → day 2° stress (MVA)
  + stiffness

LB Ⓟ L interm. 1-3 hrs. stood in line for over 1 hr. (MVA)

AGGRAVATING / RELIEVING CIRCUMSTANCES REGARDING ACTIVITIES OF DAILY LIVING

A: any activity sustained over time

R: stretching , mild exercise , hot tub , Ⓜ
(note: still unable to run)

O — HYPERTONICITIES-INTENSITY, VISUAL / PALPABLE OBSERVATIONS, ADDITIONAL TESTS

HT L BL scal., scms, traps, pecs , erec. , mass.
  Ⓛ QL , ext. rot. , psoas

Adh. + TP scms , lev scap , trap , QL

TREATMENT GOALS

↓ Adh. ↑ Rom ↑ strength ↓ posture comp. ↓ TP

MASSAGE FB SW Ⓜ

Prone:
  Back- DT w/ ROM erec. , lats
    DP/TP , XFF piri , QL

Supine:
  Neck - MET lat flex + rot
    XFF scal. DP scm
    traction

A — CHANGES DUE TO MASSAGE

↑ Rom lat flex P-cerv
↑ strength flex + ext. cerv.
↓ HT neck MΔ back LΔ psoas ∅
↓ Adh ↓ TP
Posture Δ WNL

P — SUGGESTED TREATMENT PLAN

psoas

2x mth X 2mths per 'script.

HOMEWORK

gradual ↑ activity ref: P.T.

BHW , LMP

X ADHESION	O PAIN	↻ ROTATION	
↺ TRIGGER POINT	☼ INFLAMATION	/ ELEVATION	
• TENDER POINT	≈ SPASM	≡ HYPERTONICITY	

RANGE OF MOTION			ACTIVE	
*No Right or Left evaluation	ROM		PAIN	
SPINAL	R	L	R	L
TRUNK SIDEBENDING				
TRUNK ROTATION				
EXTENSION *				
FLEXION *				

NAME **Ms. Ideal Client** DATE **1·22·93**

KEY			
WNL	Within Normal Limits	↑	Hypermobility
L	Mild	↓	Hypomobility
M	Moderate	P	Pain
S	Severe	ⓟ	No Pain

RANGE OF MOTION	ACTIVE				PASSIVE				RESISTED			
	ROM		PAIN		ROM		PAIN		STRENGTH		PAIN	
HIP	R	L	R	L	R	L	R	L	R	L	R	L
FLEXION												
EXTENSION												
ABDUCTION												
ADDUCTION												
INTERNAL ROTATION												
EXTERNAL ROTATION												
NECK	R	L	R	L	R	L	R	L	R	L	R	L
FLEXION *	WNL		⊖		WNL+		L		WNL		⊖	
EXTENSION *	WNL		⊖		WNL-		⊖		WNL		⊖	
LATERAL FLEXION	↓L	↓L	⊖	⊖	↓L	↓L	L	L	↓L	↓L	⊖	⊖
ROTATION	WNL	WNL	⊖	⊖	↑L	↑L	L	L	WNL	WNL	⊖	⊖
SHOULDER	R	L	R	L	R	L	R	L	R	L	R	L
FLEXION												
EXTENSION												
ABDUCTION												
ADDUCTION												
HORIZONTAL ADDUCTION												
HORIZONTAL ABDUCTION												
INTERNAL ROTATION												
EXTERNAL ROTATION												
PAINFUL ARC												
KNEE	R	L	R	L	R	L	R	L	R	L	R	L
FLEXION												
EXTENSION												
INTERNAL ROTATION												
EXTERNAL ROTATION												
VALGUS												
VARUS												
ANTERIOR DRAWER												
POSTERIOR DRAWER												
ANKLE	R	L	R	L	R	L	R	L	R	L	R	L
DORSIFLEXION												
PLANTARFLEXION												
INVERSION												
EVERSION												
SUPINATION												
PRONATION												
ADDUCTION												
ABDUCTION												
OTHER	R	L	R	L	R	L	R	L	R	L	R	L